The Alkalir book

your health

understand your PH level how it works and what to eat to keep your body healthy

Author by Ryan prince

Table of Contents

Introduction

congratulation on taking responsibility and full control of your health. If you think back to chemistry class, you may recall comparing an acid base, or the importance of PH balance. PH is the measure of the acidity or alkalinity of a solution. You hear about pH balance all the time, but what the heck does it mean anyway? Without getting too technical on you, pH, which stands for potential of hydrogen, measures the acid or alkaline levels of a solution. health is a treasure. of all temporal possessions it is the most precious. knowledge must be gained in regard to how to eat, and drink, and so as to preserve health. sickness is cause by violating the laws of health: I have been shown that the principles that were given us in the early days of the message are as important and should be regarded just as conscientiously today as they were then. there are some who have never followed the principles given on the question of diet. It is now time to take the light from under the bushel, and let it shine forth in clear bright ray. The principles of healthful living mean a great deal to us individually and as a people... only when we are intelligent in regard to the principles of healthful living, Can we be fully aroused to see the evils resulting from improper diet. Those who, after seeing their mistakes, have courage to change their habits will find that the reformatory process requires a struggle and much perseverance; but when correct taste are once formed they will realize that the use of the food which they formerly regarded as harmful, was slowly but surely laying the foundation for dyspepsia and other disease. It is of great importance that individually we act well on our part, and have an intelligent understanding of what we should eat and drink, and how we should live to preserve health. What you eat is closely linked to your health. Balanced nutrition has many benefits. By making healthier food choices, you can prevent or treat some conditions. These include heart disease, stroke, and diabetes. A healthy diet can help you lose weight and lower your cholesterol, and help balance up your PH level. Our bodies live and die at the cellular level. The billions of cells in our bodies must maintain alkalinity, in order to function and stay alive. The first line of defense against disease is a proper pH balance. Disease can only grow in an acidic body, which makes a condition favorable for the growth of bacteria, yeast, fungus, mold, viruses, and any other unwanted organisms. Cancer always strikes those with an over-acidic body.

Chapter 1

our health

If you have taken basic biology lesson, you will know that cells require certain conditions to function normally. Temperature and pH must be precisely engineered in order to support simple life. Our body, though it seems sturdy and above this law, it is of no different. It requires basic conditions in order to have optimal performance.

When our human body is functioning at its optimal level, human body fluids and tissues exist in a slightly alkaline state (not acidic). The food we eat often becomes the raw material to rebuild its tissue. Our PH balance can quickly become unbalanced if our diet consists largely of "acidifying" foods.

The diet of our ancestors is completely different from what we are so accustomed to these days. With the advancement of technology, the types of foods we consume are dragged along. A trip to the grocery store will shock you with aisles and aisles of processed food items and animal products. You will not have a hard time finding fast food when eating out as practically every corner of the street has one.

Even fad diets are partly to blame, for introducing a whole new eating habit, such as high-protein diets. In the recent years, consumption of animal products and refined food items has increased, as more and more people leave out the daily supply of fruits and vegetables in their diet. It comes as no surprise why, these days, many are suffering from different types of allergies, bone diseases, heart problems and many others. Some health experts link these diseases to the type of foods we eat. There are certain types of food that disrupts a certain balance in our body that, during such instance, health problems arise. If only we could modify our eating habits, it's not unlikely that prevention of diseases and restoration of health is achieved.

The body includes a number of organ systems that are adept at neutralizing and eliminating excess acid, but there is a limit to how much acid even a healthy body can cope with effectively. The body is capable of maintaining an acid-alkaline balance provided that the organs are functioning properly, that a well-balanced alkaline diet is being consumed,

How do you know whether your body is acidic

and requires your attention? Here's what you are going to do today to find out whether your body is dangerously acidic..You would first need to ask yourself whether you experience any of the symptoms below.

a. Pimples & Acnes b. Agitation c. Rapid panting breath d. Rapid heartbeat e. Muscular pain f. Pre-menstrual and menstrual cramping g. Pre-menstrual anxiety and depression h. Cold hands and feet I. Light headedness & dizziness j. Exhausted easily and low energy k. Joint pains that travel l. Food allergies m. Excessive gas n. Hyperactivity o. Lack of sex drive p. Bloating q. Heartburn & acid reflux r. Yellow & strong smelling urine s. Headaches & migraines t. Irregular heartbeat u. White coated tongue v. Hard to get up in morning w. Excess head mucous (stuffiness) If you experience more than 2 of the symptoms listed here, there is a high chance that your body is acidic and you may want to take precaution and change your diet before it accumulates and turn into deadly diseases or cancer one day. The thing is most of the people have been eating the wrong way. The 'balanced' diet that taught us about the food pyramids, balanced meal and healthy food, are the culprits in making us obese, disease, and ill. And this is because the 'balanced' diet that contains majority of meat, dairy and grains make up an acidic meal **Do you often feel out of energy especially after your meal** In fact, it is usually around 3-4 pm (depending on the time you eat your lunch) when you find yourself having difficulty in keeping yourself awake. You feel tired, exhausted and just could not continue with your work. Recently, I've read something interesting regarding this - the main reason why we experience this way is because excessive energy is needed to digest the food we ate for lunch. During 3-4 pm, our organs have already worked hard for half a day and with the excess energy needed to digest our lunch, our body naturally needs to take a rest from it. I used to assume that this is a natural process - we ought to feel lethargic in the afternoon...

But I was so wrong..

The truth is the way we eat our foods, the foods that you put into your mouths, are destructive to your body and health. For example, do you eat meat and potatoes together? How about milk and cereal, or fish and rice? Do you know that those combinations are totally destructive to your internal system and rob you of energy?

You might think that this is ridiculous..

Let me explain how these combinations are destructive and how you can save yourself large amounts of energy you may currently be wasting. Different foods are digested differently - Starchy foods require alkaline digestive medium and proteins foods like meat require and acidic medium for digestion. And when you mix both together, the medium neutralize each other. Digestion is impaired or completely arrested. This is very destructive to your body as more energy is require to digest the same amount of food. Are you as shocked as me when you first hear about this? So what can you do about it? The first step I learnt was to eat the right food and not mixing the wrong food together. For example, if I am eating starchy foods, I would not eat meat in the same meal. If I am eating meat, I would not include the starchy foods. If you are thinking whether if this is the right way, why not try it and see if you feel any difference in your body. I have tried it myself and this is the diet that not only you still can eat most of the food, but you will feel much more healthy than ever before.

What Happens When Our Body Is Acidic? To answer that, imagine your body as a receiver of different foods, and the intake of different foods, be it acidic or alkaline, will create a chemical effect that causes the overall pH of our body to fall within a scale. Being acidic means that our body's PH level is less than optimal. The optimal pH level is around 7.35-7.45, slightly alkaline. This is the best environment for our cells to function well and to fight against harmful diseases. Now, our blood creates a pH level of 7.35 – 7.45 in our body and it can hardly goes below 7.35 (but when the pH level goes below 7.35, acidosis occurs). What this means is that in order for it to remain in that alkalinity (pH of 7.35 – 7.45), to prevent acidosis from occurring, it needs to rob minerals from our bones because minerals are alkaline. That's why we get osteoporosis, that's why we get generative diseases, that's why we get tumors because the body is freaking out trying to keep the blood alkaline. **Symptoms of excess acidity** are low energy levels and constant fatigue, an excess production of mucous, nasal congestion, chronic viral diseases and infections, anxiety, stress, irritability, fragile nails, weak hair, dry skin, ovarian cysts, benign breast cysts, polycystic ovaries, headaches, arthritis, neuritis, muscle pains, hives, cramps, spasms, indigestion, and gastritis. A growing body of research suggests that having lower, or acidic, pH levels is associated with greater risk for conditions like type 2 diabetes, heart disease and obesity. The detoxifying properties of Alkaline Diets are solutions to these problems. These detoxifying properties have the ability to cleanse the blood and regenerate the cells in the body. Yeast, bacteria, fungus, and viruses need acid-based environments to thrive and multiply. However, this is not the case in Alkaline-based environments. Alkaline Diet offers to considerably lessen the chance of experiencing these problems. Food in Alkaline Diets is known for purifying the kidneys, avoiding various kidney problems. Food in the diet is a rich source of calcium, which can be a substitute to many calcium supplements. It also contains a large amount of sodium, which aids in digestion. These are but a fraction of the roles played by food in Alkaline Diets.

study that was conducted at the University of California on 9,000 women showed that those who have chronic acidosis are more prone for bone loss, as opposed to those who have normal pH levels. Scientists who conducted this experiment believe that most of the hip fractures common among middle-aged women are connected to high acidity. A diet low in vegetables and rich in animal food cause this. The reason behind this is attributed to the fact that our body borrows calcium from our bones, in order to balance PH

Balancing your pH level is far more than just choosing the alkaline foods to eat. Most people thought that just simply eating the alkaline foods would be sufficient and your pH level will return to it' optimal level.

But this is further from the truth. You would need to know exactly how to start your alkaline diet in such a way that you would absorbed all the sufficient nutrients, minerals and vitamins.

Chapter 2

What is PH level

The term PH means "potential of hydrogen" and it is used to measure the acidity of cells and other elements. The scale of acidity is measured from 0 to 14 and in the body the optimum is generally in the middle of that range. More than 90% of Americans have a pH balance that is acidic due to diet, dehydration, stress and other factors. PH is a measure of how acidic a water-based solution is. Since our bodies are mostly water, pH can be used to describe how much acid is in the fluids in our bodies. Water has a PH of 7.0. pHs lower than 7 are acidic; pHs above 7 are basic, or alkaline. Our bodies maintain our blood at a PH of about 7.4. The kidneys tightly regulate this pH balance by continuously filtering the acids and bases in the blood. The kidneys excrete just the right amount of acid or base in the urine to keep the system in pH balance. Certain other body fluids are highly acidic (like stomach acid) or basic (enzyme-rich fluids in the pancreas). These fluids are kept tightly walled off from the blood and body tissues, where they could cause damage if released inappropriately. **Digestive System** -The mouth is the entry point for food, but the digestive system often gets ready before the first piece of food even enters our mouth. How is food digested. Digestion involves the mixing of food, its movement through the digestive tract, and the chemical breakdown of the large molecules of food into smaller molecules. Digestion begins in the mouth, when we chew and swallow, and is completed in the small intestine. The digestive system consists of the parts of the body that work together to turn food and liquids into the building blocks and fuel that the body needs. Most digestive disorders, such as indigestion, nausea, bloating, gastric reflux, are symptoms caused by excess acid in the gastric region and not enough alkaline minerals in the intestinal tract. If the alkaline minerals from enzyme rich foods are missing then the pancreas will become exhausted, and once the pancreas is exhausted, it loses the ability to decode the food and tell the body what to do with it. This will lead to a degenerative spiral of entropy where organs become confused and inflamed. **Circulatory System** - Acidity is the principal cause of heart disease. It is well established that many fats are extremely important and essential for cardiovascular health. Good fats can actually help heal the inflammation that underlies arteriosclerosis. When the arteries thicken with plague it is not as a response to good fats, it is inflammation created by the internal acidic environment. The body responds to the acidity by lining the vessels with fatty plaques to prevent life-threatening leaks, which arrest imminent death, but strain the heart because the aperture for the blood to flow through is narrower. When the heart becomes completely exhausted, this is known as a heart attack. Your circulator system is a complex network of different organs and vessels that ensure proper flow of nutrients, blood, hormones and oxygen to and from cells. Your body cannot be able to maintain a healthy internal environment or fight diseases in the absence of your circulatory system. Generally, the system organs help maintain proper pH and temperature in your body to keep healthy

Your immune system is a complex network of cells that work together to protect your body against "foreign" or invading cells, including abnormal cells that can lead to cancer. Most foreign invaders are germs - infection-causing organisms that you may come into contact with, such as bad bacteria, Inside your body there is a mechanism designed to defend you from millions of bacteria, microbes, viruses, toxins and parasites While these systems protect us on a daily basis, most of us lack a working knowledge of what the immune system does and how it works. It's not important to be a scientific expert, but a brief working knowledge helps one understand inflections, the flu, colds, and other symptoms Since the immune system affects so many of our bodies' processes, it's not surprising that immune system function or dysfunction is an issue in virtually every disease. The immune system also plays a role in cancer. Since the immune system can find and attack tumor cells, when this function breaks down it can cause cancers and tumors to develop. Although scientists have learned much about the immune system, they continue to study how the body launches attacks that destroy invading microbes, infected cells, and tumors while ignoring healthy tissues. New technologies for identifying individual immune cells are now letting scientists quickly determine which targets are triggering an immune response. Improvements in microscopy are permitting the first-ever observations of B cells, T cells, and other cells as they interact within lymph nodes and other body tissues.

Immune System Protect Us Our cells have molecules on their surface called Human Leukocyte Antigens (HLA molecules) which signal to the immune system that they belong in the body. These molecules are the most variable of all human proteins, meaning that each person has a different mix that make their "HLA type" different from others. When doctors talk about transplant matches, they are really talking about matching HLA types between the donor and the recipient a difference in HLA molecules can trigger transplant rejection.

Respiratory System- Breathing is the process that brings oxygen in the air into your lungs and moves oxygen and through your body. Our lungs remove the oxygen and pass it through our bloodstream, where it's carried off to the tissues and organs that allow us to walk, talk, and move. Our lungs also take carbon dioxide from our blood and release it into the air when we breathe out. When the tissues and organs are overloaded by acidity the transport of oxygen is strangled. This suffocation means the cells cannot breathe properly. Every cell in our body needs to breathe new oxygen and to clear acidic carbon dioxide to function correctly. When the ratio of acidity is too high then wastes in the form of mucus and infections and viruses build up in our lungs, which leads to colds, bronchitis, asthma.

Arthritis -Arthritis is classified as one of the rheumatic diseases. These are conditions that are different individual illnesses, with differing features, treatments, complications, and prognosis. They are similar in that they have a tendency to affect the joints, muscles, ligaments, cartilage, and tendons, and many have the potential to affect internal body areas as well. The two main form of arthritis are Rheumatoid and Osteoarthritis. Both forms are related to pH imbalance and accumulation of acid deposits in the joints and wrists. It is this accumulated acid that damages cartilage. When the cells that produce the lubricating synovial fluids and bursa fluids are acidic, this condition causes a dryness that irritates and swells the joints. these conditions can be reverse with a proper alkaline- diet **Integumentary system** Commonly known as the skin. When the body's pH is out of balance then the buildup of acid causes inflammation and the skin is less able to function as a natural barrier against infection. Integumentary System consists of the largest organ in the body, which is the skin. This extraordinary organ system protects the internal structures of the body from damage, prevents dehydration, stores fat, and produces vitamins and hormones. It also helps to maintain homeostasis within the body by assisting in the regulation of body temperature and water balance. The integumentary system is the body's first line of defense against bacteria, viruses, and other pathogens. It also helps to provide protection from harmful ultraviolet radiation. The skin is a sensory organ in that it has receptors for detecting heat and cold.

Nervous System The nervous system is a complex collection of nerves and specialized cells known as neurons that transmit signals between different parts of the body. It is essentially the body's electrical wiring. Acidity can weakens the nervous system by depriving it of energy. This is also known as 'devitalizing' or 'enervation'. It makes the physical, mental, and emotional body weak.

The excretory system is a passive biological system that removes excess, unnecessary materials from the body fluids of an organism, The excretory system is a close partner with both the circulatory and endocrine system. The circulatory system connection is obvious. Blood that circulates through the body passes through one of the two kidneys. Urea, uric acid, and water are removed from the blood and most of the water is put back into the system The kidneys perform the task of filtering fluids and purifying our blood. If the body is overwhelmed by excess acids, compensatory mechanisms spring into action, one of them is the pulling of alkaline minerals from your bones and dumping them in the blood. If this occurs frequently enough, the minerals build up in the kidneys in the form of painful kidney stones.

Muscular System Many cells are specialised. They have structures that are adapted for their function. For example, muscle cells bring parts of the body closer together. They contain protein fibers that can contract when energy is available, making the cells shorter. There are three types of muscle Only skeletal muscles are voluntary, meaning you can control them consciously. Smooth and cardiac muscles act involuntarily.Each muscle type in the muscular system has a specific purpose. You're able to walk because of your skeletal muscles. You can digest because of your smooth muscles. And your heart beats because of your cardiac muscle. The different muscle types also work together to make these functions possible. For instance, while you're running (using skeletal muscles), your heart pumps harder (due to the cardiac muscle), which causes you to breathe heavier (using smooth muscles). There are many more diseases and disorders that are associated with an acidic condition - cataracts, osteoporosis, gout, cancer, migraines, constipation, morning sickness, stroke, allergies, diabetes, obesity, etc. With this awareness of how acidity affects us, we can all choose to make informed and healthy decisions to what we put in our diet to keep our body healthy.

Do PH really that dangerous?

Yes, indeed it is! Nothing does well in an overly acidic or alkaline pH medium, least of all the human body! Just as acid rain can destroy a forest and alkaline wastes can pollute a lake, an imbalanced pH continuously corrodes all body tissue, slowly eating into the 60,000 miles of our veins and arteries like corrosives eating into marble. If left unchecked, an imbalanced pH will interrupt all cellular activities and functions, from the beating of your heart to the neural firing of your brain... An imbalanced pH interferes with all life itself!

Your body must maintain its internal PH within a very narrow range. A healthy body maintains adequate alkaline reserves to balance the acids in order to maintain this PH. When excess acids must be neutralized our alkaline reserves are depleted leaving the body in a weakened condition. A PH balanced diet, according to many experts, is a vital key to maintaining the reserves necessary for health maintenance. It is recommended that you test your PH levels to determine if your body's PH needs immediate attention. By using PH test strips, you can determine your pH factor quickly and easily in the privacy of your own home. If your urinary PH fluctuates between 6.0 to 6.5 in the morning and between 6.5 and 7.0 in the evening, your body is functioning within a healthy range. If your saliva stays between 6.5 and 7.5 all day, your body is functioning within a healthy range. The best time to test your PH is about one hour before a meal and two hours after a meal. PH of the body's fluids Water is the most abundant compound in the human body, comprising 70% of the body. The body has an acid-alkaline (or acid-base) ratio called the PH which is a balance between positively charged ions (acid-forming) and negatively charged ions (alkaline-forming.) The body continually strives to balance PH. When this balance is compromised many problems can occur. the lower the PH the more acidic the solution, the higher the PH the more alkaline the solution. When a solution is neutral it is neither acid nor alkaline and has a PH of 7.

What affects PH?

The consumption of too little water is a common source of weakness and fatigue. Drinking water will perk you up just as a wilted flower perks up in water. To understand how water can help give you a midday boost...all you have to do is understand how your body's PH level works. Normally, the kidneys maintain our electrolyte levels, those of calcium, magnesium, potassium and sodium. When we are exposed to acidic substances, these electrolytes are used to combat acidity. High degrees of acidity force our bodies to rob minerals from the bones, cells, organs and tissues. Cells end up lacking enough minerals to properly dispose of waste or oxygenate completely. Vitamin absorption is compromised by mineral loss. Toxins and pathogens accumulate in the body and the immune system becomes suppressed.

The blood PH has a serious effect on all of the body's systems and the body uses different mechanisms to control the blood's acid-base balance. The blood's acid-base balance is controlled by the body because even minor deviations from the normal range can severely affect the brain, arteries, the heart, muscles, and many organs. It can contribute to overwhelming the body leading to serious disease such as cancer. Most diets cause an unhealthy Acid PH. In fact, diet appears to be the major influence in maintaining appropriate PH levels throughout the body. Research demonstrates that when food is metabolized and broken down, it leaves certain chemical and metallic residues, a noncombustible "ash" which, when combined with our body fluids, yields either acid or alkali potentials of PH. Certain foods are "acid-forming" in nature, whereas others are known to be "alkali-forming." **acid-forming and alkaline-forming.** Most high protein foods (such as meat, fish, poultry and eggs), nearly all carbohydrates (including grains, breads and pastas) and fats are "acid-forming." And most fruits and vegetables are "alkaline-forming." Although citrus fruits, such as oranges and grapefruit, contain organic acids and may have an acid taste, they are not acid-forming when metabolized, leaving no acidic residue. Similarly, Free Form Amino Acids are not acid-forming, but instead offer unique buffering capabilities to the body to help offset acidic wastes. The length of time you can hold your breath is one technique you can use to document the difference that occurs after adapting a more alkaline-producing diet. Watching your diet can help. If you're too acid, increase the number of fruits and vegetables you eat. If you're too alkaline, increase the amounts of acid-forming foods consumed. You may want to consider a water system that simultaneously filters your tap water and creates alkaline water. High levels of lead in drinking water is a primary concern of PH. It places adults at risk for health problems such as cancer, stroke, kidney disease, memory problems and high blood pressure. Children are at a greater risk because their rapidly growing bodies absorb the contaminant more quickly.

So, what does PH mean for water? Basically, the PH value is a good indicator of whether water is hard or soft. The PH of pure water is 7. In general, water with a PH lower than 7 is considered acidic, and with a PH greater than 7 is considered basic. The normal range for PH in surface water systems is 6.5 to 8.5, and the PH range for groundwater systems is between 6 to 8.5. Alkalinity is a measure of the capacity of the water to resist a change in PH that would tend to make the water more acidic. The measurement of alkalinity and PH is needed to determine the corrosiveness of the water.

Copper, Iron, Zinc and Manganese are also classified as secondary drinking water contaminants. These contaminants are likely to cause hard water and staining problems at home. But if found in elevated levels, they could cause a variety of health issues. That includes nausea, vomiting, diarrhea, stomach cramps, kidney disease, liver disease.

PH related to Teeth and Gums

There are many benefits to eating an alkaline diet. Over-acidity in the body can result in chronic health issues, while an alkaline diet can help to prevent these same problems. Some of the symptoms of an over-acid diet include fatigue, gum and teeth problems, a tendency towards getting sick frequently, pain and inflammation, and premature aging When the PH level of the body is too acidic, it stands to reason that the mouth will also be quite acidic. Unfortunately, when the level of acid in the mouth is too high, it can cause bacteria to grow at a much faster rate. Bacteria can cause a number of different problems in the mouth, such as gum disease and bad breath. A high level of acid and bacteria in the mouth will also increase a person's chances for tooth decay. Many people note an improvement in their overall level of oral health after switching to a diet program that promotes an alkaline pH level in the body. Vitamin-rich foods. Foods containing calcium — such as cheese, almonds and leafy greens and foods high in phosphorous — such as meat, eggs and fish can help keep tooth enamel strong and healthy, according to the American Dental Association Swap out soda with water. When you eat sugary foods or sip sugary drinks for long periods of time, plaque bacteria use that sugar to produce acids that attack your enamel, the hard surface of your tooth. Most carbonated soft drinks, including diet soda, are acidic and therefore, bad for your teeth. Caffeinated beverages, such as colas can also dry out your mouth. If you do consume soft drinks, try to rinse with water. Before your next sip, check the label to make sure your drink of choice is low in sugar or drink water.

 Particularly important is calcium, which helps to form strong teeth and bones, and vitamin D, which the body needs to absorb calcium. You need lots of calcium for healthy teeth and gums

Adding more vegetables to our diet is one of the most important things we can do for our health, both general and dental. Our bodies need nutrients to operate at peak performance. Vitamin and mineral deficiencies are linked to many serious health conditions. Without the proper vitamins and minerals, our immune systems are weakened and do not have the ability to fight off bacteria and infections. While some vegetables are acidic, many vegetables are alkaline so they will help neutralize the PH in the mouth and the body.

The PH of your Saliva

 A low PH of your saliva signifies an acidic environment. People with acidic saliva often experience dental problems as a result of their own saliva damaging their teeth. They may wonder why no amount of brushing or flossing prevents cavities, or why they suffer from broken restorations, gum recession or sensitivity. One solution is to bring the PH of the saliva to a more alkaline state. But how much more of the alkaline-producing foods should we have and how much less of the acid-producing foods is ideal? Of course, you can check your own PH level or ask a doctor to do it for you. If you want to do it yourself, you can place a litmus strip under your tongue. The color of the strip will change according to the acidity level from your saliva, after which you can match the color to the color on the chart that comes with the litmus strips.

Signs that you may be acidic There are likewise telltale signs in your body that reveal how much of those acid-forming meats and sweets you should "cut back" on. These are uncomfortable and painful signs that appear as weight gain, joint pains, heartburn, poor digestion (irregular bowel movement and intestinal cramping), fatigue, muscle weakness, urinary tract problems, receding gums, kidney stones, bone loss and skin problems. If you have three or more of these symptoms, then it may be time to shift to an alkaline diet. For example, many people think of lemons as acidic, and while they are classified as an acidic fruit, lemons are actually an alkaline forming food. During the process of digestion the acids are oxidized into carbon dioxide and water, therefore they do not create an acid condition in the system. Calcium, iron, magnesium, potassium, and sodium are the main alkalizing minerals. Foods that are high in these minerals are considered alkaline forming foods. Most foods have both acid and alkaline minerals in them, so those with greater concentrations of acidic minerals are considered acidic and vice versa.

If weight loss is your goal, you don't have to look far for a plan guaranteed to work. Diet pills, meal replacements and food-specific diets make promises that often fail to live up to the hype. The most successful weight-loss plan incorporates commitment, healthy eating habits and exercise. It can be helpful in achieving your goals to understand how factors such blood PH affect the weight-loss equation.

In order to lose 1 pound a week, you must reduce your calorie intake by 3,500 calories, burn the equivalent of 3,500 calories through exercise or use a combination of both methods. Keeping weight off requires striking a balance between the calories you consume and the calories you burn. Blood PH, or the acid-base balance in your blood, plays a role in weight loss and determines how you burn fat. If the foods you eat upset this balance, weight loss becomes difficult or impossible.   **Vaginal PH:** what even is it? Well, you may remember from chemistry that the PH of something determines how acidic or basic it is, and you might be surprised to learn that the PH of a women vagina directly relates to how healthy it is. A healthy vaginal PH is somewhere between 3.5 to 4.5, and if you're healthy it should regulate itself and keep it in this acidic range. When your PH is unhealthy, you will likely notice an unpleasant odor, which is a sign of an imbalance like a yeast infection or bacterial vaginosis. A slightly acidic vagina is the perfect environment for the types of good bacteria that help keep your vagina clean and healthy – and most harmful bacteria have a hard time surviving in an acidic environment. Keeping those harmful bacteria at bay is not only important for general hygiene and comfort, but also to help avoid infection and diseases. A PH level above 4.5 can make you more susceptible to vaginitis, or inflammation of the vaginal tissue, which can be caused by infections like yeast and bacterial vaginosis.

Vaginal Health is one of the most important component of overall women health. Your vagina is a pretty amazing part of your anatomy. Not only does it bring pleasure, it also helps you create and bring life into the world. Add to that its ability to keep itself clean, and you have one extraordinary body part. The vagina cleans itself by secreting natural fluids and maintaining a healthy PH to encourage the growth of good bacteria and discourage harmful bacteria from taking up residence. Adding coconut oil down there doesn't only your vagina more lubricated, but its anti-fungal and anti-bacterial properties do a great job at preventing yeast infections. Balancing your diet in general and including things like pineapples, strawberries, yogurt, soy (the list goes on!) can influence your PH balance in positive ways. Beverages like water, cranberry juice and pineapple juice are also proven to improve vaginal health, and keep it moist and hydrated. your diet can increase the amount of good bacteria in your vagina called lactobacillus. So, eat healthy, and your vagina will thank you!

Chapter 3

Alkalinize Cold Sores and Stress

A statistic that may amaze you is that almost 90% of the world's population has the herpes simplex virus. However, only a small percentage of adults complain about and seek treatment for this virus from their doctor. There are a variety of medications on the market which can provide temporary relief. Tablets are often prescribed by the doctors. Creams are also prescribed which, if applied according to the specified directions, can treat your HSV - 1 virus externally. These creams, tablets, etc can provide you with temporary relief but for permanent relief you need to use both traditional and non - traditional approaches.

The PH level in your body should be close to the normal level which is 7.0 and above. There are many other factors which can prevent your body from being in the normal PH range. Unhealthy food habits and stress can increase acidity in your body and make you susceptible to all kinds of diseases. Lack of oxygen or oxygen deficient bodies are highly prone to diseases. The herpes simplex virus is anaerobic and it cannot survive in the presence of oxygen. There are numerous ways by which you can increase oxygen content levels in your body. Exercise is a cost effective manner of increasing oxygen levels in your body. Exercise in the early morning hours is recommended because air has comparatively high levels of oxygen. Exercise should be done systematically so that your body works every muscle group. This should improve the oxygen flow in your body.

Exercise should be done with frequent breaks in between so as not to add stress on your body, rather than relieve it. Excessive exercise increases the acidity of your body due to lactic acid build up. Stress is another very important factor which weakens the body, making it susceptible to disease. Stress and tension will increase the acidity of your system. Stress releases many different types of acids and harmful chemicals tin an attempt to cope with the situation you are in. This is of course useful if you are running away from a lion or escaping from a burning building. However, chronic stress is very hard on the body and increases the acidity content in your system.

Herpes simplex virus thrives in acidic and less oxygenated bodies and its attacks are frequent in when your body is in such a situation. The human body is a precise machine and it needs to be maintained using common sense and listening to what it is telling you.

Alkalinize Your Body to Cure Your Cold Sores Through Water

How wonderful it would be if we had a permanent cure for cold sores. A Cold sore or fever blister is technically known as the Herpes Simplex Virus type 1 (HSV-1). If you are in some fantasy world thinking that by the use of medications you can cure the cold sores virus permanently then you are fooling yourself. There is no medication available today which says that it can cure this virus permanently. The only option available for you is to cure it from both inside and outside of your body.

Stress is the main cause of diseases worldwide. Herpes simplex virus gets triggered when your body is under chronic stressed causing your immune system to weaken and fail to combat the virus. Doctors have recommended different types of foods such as Lysine. Lysine is an amino acid which combats the virus and decrease the number of outbreaks. Lysine can be found in various types of foods such as potatoes, fish, chicken, beans, etc. Generally the required amount of intake might not be greater than what you can get from these foods and so many doctors also prescribe supplements.

Alkalinity of the body is the decisive factor in maintaining human wellness. The human body needs to be alkaline to fight many types of diseases and viruses. Many people fail to understand that by changing their diet habits and unhealthy lifestyle they can put this herpes simplex virus into remission. Water offers a cheap and effective solution to maintain normal alkaline level. There are certain products such as water Oz alkalizer which increases the alkalinity of water, which you can take to help increase your PH levels thus bringing your body to a stable and healthy alkaline state. Water flushes out waste products in our body and carries essential minerals, nutrients, etc throughout the body. Drinking plenty of water makes your system stable and healthier. There are many products on the shelf which are effective in increasing pH levels such as Water OZ Body alkalizer. This product can also be used in acidic foods such as lemon, orange juice, etc to reduce acidity.

Alkalinize Your Body to Cure Cold Sores With The Right Nutrition

Cold sores can be detected early if you can make yourself aware of the warning signs. Common signals such as tingling, itching and warmth at the point of occurrence should be an indicator of cold sore developing. This phase lasts for several hours and is the best time to take precautions. During this phase the infected area should not be touched. Touching or itching will act as a catalyst for the virus to spread to other parts. In case you want to touch, it would be advisable to clean the surface with anti - bacterial agent and then wipe it with cotton.

Nutrition plays a very important role in making the herpes simplex virus dormant. Good exercise and dietary habits need to be followed if you want to make the virus dormant. It is very important to understand that simple slight changes in food habits will improve the alkaline content in your body thus making the virus dormant for very long periods, if not the rest of your life.

The herpes simplex virus needs an acidic climate to thrive and multiply. A balanced dietary approach between acidic and alkaline foods will help you in getting the much needed respite from herpes simplex virus type 1. Diet restriction is very important because it can actually make the virus dormant. Do consult a nutritionist before taking any advice.

if you experience cold sores some of the food you need avoid

Pork, shellfish, margarine products, artificial sweeteners, junk food, mayonnaise, caffeine, MSG, high fat dairy products, alcohol, saturated fat foods, etc. Chocolates should be completely avoided by people suffering from the herpes simplex virus. This virus can also get triggered from artificial sweeteners because of the chemicals and various kinds of preservatives used in them.

Foods which have a high fiber content are good for the heart and also for the increasing metabolism. Care should be taken to avoid acidic foods when you are suffering from herpes simplex virus. Juices, water and milk are the best ways to stay healthy and fit. Caffeine can be consumed in a limited quantity if you are in the habit of drinking it a lot and smoking should be totally avoided.

Oxygen As we know, humans need oxygen for basic bodily functions. Oxygen contains certain properties which help in metabolism. Without these basic functions the human body cannot continue to live. Lack of oxygen in the blood cells causes diseases to be able to run rampant. Disease causing bacteria and virus tend to survive in conditions where there is low amount of oxygen. Herpes simplex virus type 1 cannot be destroyed by increasing the amount of oxygen levels in the body but it can be made dormant.

Oxygen supplements are generally recommended by doctors all over the world. Alternate medicine consultants also recommend medications and oxygen supplement drops. These oxygen supplement drops are easily absorbed by the body due to their fluid state. These drops are available in pharmacies and from chemists and over the internet as over the counter drugs. Increased levels of nascent oxygen is very helpful for other body process such as digestion, increased levels of energy, blood flow, immune system, etc. Oxygen is a free radical scavenger and it is known to cure many disease caused by anaerobic bacteria in the body without damaging the tissue and aerobic bacteria. Oxygen supplement drops do not have any smell and they do not tend to cause a nauseous feeling. **battle Cold Sores from The Outside** A cold sore can be very embarrassing because it affects the most visible parts of the body such as lips, mouth, nostrils, eye lids, etc. During those 9 - 12 days in which the cold sore is present, it passes through various stages of developments. These stages can cause pain and swelling. These blisters grow in size and then ultimately after the prolonged cycle they dry up. Care should be taken when a cold sore dries up as it may leave a mark or a dark spot. These are some of the precautions which you can take to battle the herpes simplex virus from outside.

Affected part should be cleaned with an anti bacterial agent and then later cleaned thoroughly with cotton. Itching, pain and swelling are three common stages of this bacteria during which you should resist the urge to itch or touch the affected part. If you happen to touch it make sure that you clean your hand thoroughly with an anti - bacterial agent to prevent the spread to other parts of your body and to other people.

So, as we mentioned, the first thing you need to do is clean it up with anti - bacterial agent and then later apply Zinc or DMSO at the affected part. Protamine zinc will help you achieve a very fast recovery. Generally it is estimated that protamine zinc speeds up the recovery process up to 30%.

A cold sore takes 9-12 days before entering into the remission phase where the virus becomes dormant. These blisters are known to create emotional problems because of its constant reappearance and the visibility of the sore. There are cures which make the visible blisters dormant. If you are affected right now it is important that you seek medical advice and get treated for the cold sore. It is very important to learn the basic nature and structure of the virus to combat it effectively from inside and outside of the human body.

Humans suffer from cold sores because of unhealthy life styles, oxygen deficient bodies, acidity, stress and strain, and excessive exposure to sun, consumption of junk food, chocolates, poor immune system, etc. The immune system should be strengthened from the inside to combat this virus effectively. The immune system can be improved if you practice healthy habits such as avoiding junk food, reducing smoking and drinking (alcohol), etc. White blood cells in your body are the primary defense against all viruses and diseases small and large (even cancer). Exercising your body helps it stays in shape and also improves your metabolism and improves the oxygen level in your body.

Lower levels of oxygen in their system tend to trigger diseases. This lower level of oxygen gives rise to acid levels in the human body. This acidic nature of the human body is the appropriate climate for the herpes simplex virus.

The herpes simplex virus is anaerobic and thrives in acidic climates with low oxygen levels. Improving oxygen content in the human body stabilizes the whole system and maintains PH level which is very essential for the body to operate smoothly. In previous times oxygen levels in the atmosphere were around 40% which has gradually gotten reduced to 20%. There are certain oxygen supplements such as water Oz which helps in increasing the nascent oxygen levels inside the human body. Oxygen supplements such as water Oz releases molecular oxygen upon coming into contact with the stomach acids.

Oxygen stabilizers work so well because of the "enzyme enhancing" qualities of the chlorite ion. Chlorite ion contains molecules of chlorine and oxygen with a strong negative charge. Chlorine dioxide is also a potent oxidizer and a killer of microbes. Chlorite is very helpful in cell oxidation.

Vitamin C with bioflavonoid can be an effective combatant against virus. These nutrients and vitamins strengthen the immune system. Care should be taken not to take more than the recommended dose of any medication even if it is a vitamin. Consult your doctor for advice.

Two things need to be done in regards to your immune system; one is strengthening the immune system so that it effectively combats virus and destroys the cells causing the virus. Secondly you need to stop the virus from replicating. If we can destroy and stop the virus from replicating then we can put the virus into a dormant state. Exercise and eating habits need to be changed to effectively combat the virus. Nascent oxygen is very much required to combat the diseases and viruses present in your body.

Alkaline food can protect you from many diseases and can increase the immune response of the body. There are many reasons for the virus attacks such as a weak immune system, unhealthy lifestyle, lower levels of oxygen inside the body, acidity (PH below 7), etc. Alkalinity of the body should be maintained at any cost because acidity will make your body susceptible to diseases. A balanced diet which contains acidic and alkaline food is best for the body.

Acidic foods are also useful to avoid certain kinds of diseases but anything more than the normal can play havoc. Fruits and vegetables should be your ideal choice. Vegetables and fruits which contain vitamins, enzymes, minerals, water, fiber, importantly antioxidants, etc should be consumed.

You might not be able to get all these essential dietary requirements in one day but you can plan out a course of diet with your nutritionist who can help you chart out the diet plan. Alkaline foods should be 75% of your meal and also don't forget to include some essential fruits which could restore your energy.

Chapter 4

Why we need iodine

Iodine is an element found mainly in seawater and in soil close to the sea. The human body needs iodine to make thyroid hormone. During fetal development, infancy, and childhood, thyroid hormone is essential for the brain and nervous system to develop normally. Too little iodine, and thus too little thyroid hormone, can lead to mental retardation, dwarfism, hearing loss, and other problems. Later in life, thyroid hormone controls metabolism. Adults who don't take in enough iodine can develop a goiter (a swelling of the butterfly-shaped thyroid gland in the neck), and the low output of thyroid hormone can lead to sluggish metabolism, poor thinking skills, infertility, thyroid cancer, and other conditions.

Current dietary guidelines recommend that men and women ages 19 and older get 150 micrograms of iodine a day. Women who are pregnant should get 220 micrograms, and women who are breast-feeding an infant should get 290 micrograms.

Iodine is a mineral that is needed in the diet to ensure that the thyroid works properly.

Thyroid hormones play an important role in a wide range of bodily functions, including metabolism, bone health, immune response, and development of the central nervous system (CNS). Iodine helps convert thyroid stimulating hormone (TSH) to triiodothyronine (T3) and thyroxine (T4). This conversion is important for the thyroid to function properly.

An iodine imbalance can lead to an overactive or underactive thyroid.

Around 70 to 80 percent of iodine is found in the thyroid gland in the neck. The rest is in the blood, the muscles, the ovaries, and other parts of the body.

Iodine deficiency is rare in Western nations because salt is iodized. However, an estimated 2 billion people worldwide remain at risk for iodine deficiency, and about 300 million people worldwide suffer from thyroid gland dysfunction Iodine is a mineral found in some foods. The body needs iodine to make thyroid hormones. These hormones control the body's metabolism and many other important functions. The body also needs thyroid hormones for proper bone and brain development during pregnancy and infancy.

Iodine reduces thyroid hormone and can kill fungus, bacteria, and other microorganisms such as amoebas. A specific kind of iodine called potassium iodide is also used to treat (but not prevent) the effects of a radioactive accident.

When faced with a radioactive cloud it is absolutely imperative that you take iodine, whatever iodine you can get your hands on. If the only iodine available is topical iodine that is not suitable for oral use then you should paint your body and your children's bodies with it. Few people have ready access to the Nascent iodine so will not enjoy its ease of application in repeated measured dosages that are more gentle to the system, thus yielding fewer side effects. Because Nascent is in the atomic form, it is absorbed faster and that can also be advantageous in emergency situations. Its only downside is the expense of having to use so much of it.

What happens if I don't get enough iodine

Everyone needs iodine in their diet for healthy thyroid function and a healthy metabolism. Hypothyroidism (see symptoms below) can be caused by a lack of iodine in the diet, which prevents the thyroid from making enough of the necessary hormones.

Iodine deficiency is the single most common cause of preventable mental retardation and brain damage in the world. The most alarming consequences of iodine deficiency occur during foetal and infant development. Maternal iodine deficiency may cause miscarriage, other pregnancy complications, such as premature delivery and infertility.

Thyroid hormones – and therefore iodine – are essential for normal development of the brain. If the foetus or newborn is not exposed to enough thyroid hormone, it may not survive or may have permanent mental retardation. Low birth weights may also result from iodine deficiency.

Iodine deficiency is a major cause of lowered IQ in children, according to leading international health authorities, including the World Health organization (UNICEF and the International Council for the Control of Iodine Deficiency Disorders (ICCIDD). When the deficiency is very severe, the effect can be up to 15 IQ points lower than normal (or a reduction of 15 per cent of the average IQ.

Your thyroid can hold a maximum of 50 mg of iodine

20 percent of the iodine in your body is held in your skin (if your skin is depleted of iodine, you will not be able to sweat)

32 percent of your body's iodine stores are in your muscles (if muscles are depleted, pain and other fibromyalgia symptoms.

What are some effects of iodine on health?

Scientists are studying iodine to understand how it affects health.

Fetal and infant development

Women who are pregnant or breastfeeding need to get enough iodine for their babies to grow and develop properly. Breastfed infants get iodine from breast milk. However, the iodine content of breast milk depends on how much iodine the mother gets.

To make adequate amounts of iodine available for proper fetal and infant development, several national and international groups recommend that pregnant and breastfeeding women and infants take iodine supplements. In the United States and Canada, the American Thyroid Association recommends that pregnant and breastfeeding women take prenatal vitamin/mineral supplements containing iodine (150 mcg/day). However, only about half the prenatal multivitamins sold in the United States contain iodine.

Cognitive function during childhood

Severe iodine deficiency during childhood has harmful effects on the development of the brain and nervous system. The effects of mild iodine deficiency during childhood are more difficult to measure, but mild iodine deficiency might cause subtle problems with neurological development. Giving iodine supplements to children with mild iodine deficiency improves their reasoning abilities and overall cognitive function. In children living in iodine-deficient areas, iodine supplements seem to improve both physical and mental development. More study is needed to fully understand the effects of mild iodine deficiency and of iodine supplements on cognitive function.

Radiation-induced thyroid cancer

Nuclear accidents can release radioactive iodine into the environment, increasing the risk of thyroid cancer in people who are exposed to the radioactive iodine, especially children. People with iodine deficiency who are exposed to radioactive iodine are especially at risk of developing thyroid cancer.

Deficiency Symptoms Of Iodine

A deficiency of iodine can have serious effects on the body. The symptoms of its deficiency include frustration, depression, mental retardation, poor perception levels, goiter, abnormal weight gain, decreased fertility, coarse skin, chances of stillbirth in expectant mothers, constipation, and fatigue. In severe cases, mental retardation associated with diseases such as cretinism, characterized by physical malformations, can be the result. According to WHO reports, this deficiency is one of the leading causes of mental retardation all over the world.

Detoxes Fluoride

You don't want to consumer too much Iodine just to try to get rid of fluoride, but getting the right amount of Iodine will help to make sure that your body has the ability to combat the level of toxic fluoride. Fluoride accumulates in the body over time, so it's good to be able to help neutralize it with Iodine, rather than letting it store up over several months of even years. The good news is that you are likely getting enough Iodine, so this is happening for most people automatically.

Improves Metabolism

Your thyroid is a major factor in regulating your metabolism, and if your Iodine levels are low, you run the risk of having an underactive thyroid, and therefore a sluggish metabolism. Get your Iodine levels to a good place and all else being equal you should see an increase in your metabolic rate. It's always a good idea to get tested to see if you do indeed have an Iodine deficiency, rather than just assuming you do and taking a supplement when it's not needed.

Protects Thyroid Because of the world we live in, each day we're bombarded by products, foods, drinks, and lifestyles that expose us to free radicals. These attack the body, including the thyroid. Having the right amount of Iodine helps to protect the thyroid from free radical damage. Not having enough means you are leaving it susceptible to this damage, which over time can lead to additional problems and conditions. **Balances Hormones** Having low amounts of Iodine can throw your hormones out of whack because it has a direct effect on your thyroid gland, which in turn regulates many of your hormones. It has also been said to help bring your libido up to its natural levels. Sometimes it can be hard to identify the symptoms of low Iodine, but together with your doctor you can figure it out, and if you find out that you've been running a shortage you can take steps to make things right again.

Improves Hair Growth

You shouldn't start taking massive amounts of Iodine in hopes that it will help turn around your male pattern baldness, but it has been linked to the health of the hair, and how fast it grows. This is just one sign that you may be running behind on your Iodine, if you've noticed that your hair is not growing as quickly, or as fully as it used to. Be sure to look for other signs before drawing conclusions.

Increases Energy Levels

Not getting enough Iodine each day sets you up for not having as much energy as you would otherwise. This is because it helps with proper thyroid function, and this is a big factor in whether you feel up and ready to go, or if you feel lethargic and like you need more rest. It's not something that is often discussed when talking about healthy energy levels, but more and more we're finding out the important role that Iodine plays in that department.

Provides Protection from Radiation

One benefit of Iodine that most people will hopefully not need to experience is that it helps protect from radiation. This can come in handy for disasters like the one at the nuclear power plant in Japan, but doctors are also using it to help patients recover from radiation treatments.

Protects from Pathogens Iodine is being considered more and more as an alternative to using antibiotics in the body to treat certain pathogens. Many people do not like the idea of taking an oral antibiotic, since it's been known to kill off good bacteria as well as bad, and can leave the body with excess levels of Candida. But Iodine has been shown to have a similar effect while not damaging healthy bacteria that the body needs.

Protects Against Cancer

In a process known as apoptosis, Iodine helps the body kill off cells that could end up leading to cancer. This is one of the most important reasons to get your Iodine levels checked at your next doctor visit, or even to schedule a particular visit to have all of your vitamin and mineral levels checked. You can't really know what you need to focus on if you don't know what you're lacking.

Chapter 5

balance your PH to heal your body

Digestive System

Most digestive disorders, such as indigestion, nausea, bloating, gastric reflux, are symptoms caused by excess acid in the gastric region and not enough alkaline minerals in the intestinal tract. If the alkaline minerals from enzyme rich foods are missing then the pancreas will become exhausted, and once the pancreas is exhausted, it loses the ability to decode the food and tell the body what to do with it. This will lead to a degenerative spiral of entropy where organs become confused and inflamed

Digestive System

Most digestive disorders, such as indigestion, nausea, bloating, gastric reflux, are symptoms caused by excess acid in the gastric region and not enough alkaline minerals in the intestinal tract. If the alkaline minerals from enzyme rich foods are missing then the pancreas will become exhausted, and once the pancreas is exhausted, it loses the ability to decode the food and tell the body what to do with it. This will lead to a degenerative spiral of entropy where organs become confused and inflamed.

Circulatory System Acidity is the principal cause of heart disease. It is well established that many fats are extremely important and essential for cardiovascular health. Good fats can actually help heal the inflammation that underlies arteriosclerosis. When the arteries thicken with plague it is not as a response to good fats, it is inflammation created by the internal acidic environment. The body responds to the acidity by lining the vessels with fatty plaques to prevent life-threatening leaks, which arrest imminent death, but strain the heart because the aperture for the blood to flow through is narrower. When the heart becomes completely exhausted, this is known as a heart attack.

Immune System

Acidic environments are breeding grounds for anaerobic pathogens whereas the high levels hydrogen of rich body fluids keep bad bacteria inactive. As the great scientist, Antoine Béchamp famously observed 'The germ is nothing, the terrain is everything.' Whether bad bacteria and pathogens incubate or remain dormant, all depends on the ratio of cellular PH.

The germ theory is a narrow view that has been adopted by the current medical establishment, which conveniently relies on a profitable cut, burn, and poison approach to sickness. Surgery, radiation, and pharmaceutical drugs are an invasive approach that is ineffective because they works against the body's natural functions to heal itself, and it fails to address the underlying cause and only treats the symptoms.

Respiratory System

When the tissues and organs are overloaded by acidity the transport of oxygen is strangled. This suffocation means the cells cannot breathe properly. Every cell in our body needs to breathe new oxygen and to clear acidic carbon dioxide to function correctly. When the ratio of acidity is too high then wastes in the form of mucus and infections and viruses build up in our lungs, which leads to colds, bronchitis, asthma, etc.

Skeletal System

Arthritis is one of the most disabling diseases in developed countries. The word arthritis means "inflammation of the joint" and is used to describe pain, stiffness, and swelling in the joints. The two main form of arthritis are Rheumatoid and Osteoarthritis. Both forms are related to PH imbalance and accumulation of acid deposits in the joints and wrists. It is this accumulated acid that damages cartilage. When the cells that produce the lubricating synovial fluids and bursa fluids are acidic, this condition causes a dryness that irritates and swells the joints. When uric acid builds up it tends to deposit in the form of crystals, like broken glass in the feet, hands, knees and back. Osteoarthritis is not a 'wear-and-tear' condition. Arthritis can be arrested and reversed using a specific protocol that developed using alkaline minerals.

Integumentary System

Commonly known as the skin. When the body's PH is out of balance then the buildup of acid causes inflammation and the skin is less able to function as a natural barrier against infection. As a result, the skin tends to develop lesions and sores open to the surface of the body, and the formation of skin eruptions occur like pimples or rashes.

Nervous System

Acidity weakens the nervous system by depriving it of energy. This is also known as 'devitalizing' or 'enervation'. It makes the physical, mental, and emotional body weak.

Excretory System

This is also known as the urinary system. It is made up of multiple organs, the main one being the kidneys. The kidneys perform the task of filtering fluids and purifying our blood. If the body is overwhelmed by excess acids, compensatory mechanisms spring into action, one of them is the pulling of alkaline minerals from your bones and dumping them in the blood. If this occurs frequently enough, the minerals build up in the kidneys in the form of painful kidney stones.

Muscular System When acidity increases in the muscle cells, it disrupts the metabolism breakdown of glucose and oxygen to energy. This means muscles perform poorly in an acidic environment. An alkaline system on the other hand allows for much better aerobic metabolism and energy for the body's recovery from strenuous exercise. I can often observe when someone is acidic from their breathing because they take large gulping inhales while doing the simplest tasks like walking and talking, which

suggests their body finds it difficult to adequately deliver oxygen into the cells - a symptom of acidosis.

Reproductive System

Still much research is being done to discover the exact link between sexual dysfunction and acidity and also infertility and acidity. Many health experts that claim acidity is correlated with three different disorders in reproductive health:

Decreases male and female arousal.

Decreases sexual enjoyment and particularly female satisfaction/climax.

Decreases fertility and increases the tendency to miscarry.

There are many more diseases and disorders that are associated with an acidic condition - cataracts, osteoporosis, gout, cancer, migraines, constipation, morning sickness, stroke, allergies, diabetes, obesity, etc. With this awareness of how acidity affects us, we can all choose to make informed and empowered healthy decisions for wellness and good nutrition.

Nutrition and Health Are Closely Related Over the past century, essential nutrient deficiencies have dramatically decreased, many infectious diseases have been conquered, and the majority of the U.S. population can now anticipate a long and productive life. However, as infectious disease rates have dropped, the rates of noncommunible diseases—specifically, chronic diet-related diseases—have risen, due in part to changes in lifestyle behaviors. A history of poor eating and physical activity patterns have a cumulative effect and have contributed to significant nutrition- and physical activity-related health challenges that now face the U.S. population. About half of all American adults—117 million individuals—have one or more preventable chronic diseases, many of which are related to poor quality eating patterns and physical inactivity. These include cardiovascular disease, high blood pressure, type 2 diabetes, some cancers, and poor bone health. More than two-thirds of adults and nearly one-third of children and youth are overweight or obese. These high rates of overweight and obesity and chronic disease have persisted for more than two decades and come not only with increased health risks, but also at high cost. In 2008, the medical costs associated with obesity were estimated to be $147 billion. In 2012, the total estimated cost of diagnosed diabetes was $245 billion, including $176 billion in direct medical costs and $69 billion in decreased productivity.

Chapter 6

Correcting your PH

Your PH levels are influenced by various factors. More importantly, what you put into your body affects the creation of the PH level.

Unhealthy diet, a diet too high in fatty foods, contributes for our body chemistry to become too acidic which increases the risk of illness, including cancer.

The better way to balance your PH level is to eat as clean as possible, which means to restrict yourself from processed food. Instead, consume organic foods which can reduce the number of chemicals that enter your body.

Namely, the acidic state of your body is referred to as its pH balance. It is similar to the one of a swimming pool, and if the water is with a high pH balance, it indicates that it become too alkaline and has similar effects on the human body. On the other hand, if the PH balance of a pool is low, it indicates that the water became too acidic and leads to dry itchy skin and sore, burning eyes and nose.

Proper diet is essential to restore your body's PH to homeostasis. Therefore, it is of great importance to distinguish what foods are alkaline and what are acid.

Raw vegetables are alkaline and meats are acidic, but this does not mean that you need to completely eliminate meat and eat only raw vegetables. Instead, you simply need to consume greater portions of vegetables than meat.

Non-Acidic Fruits The majority of fruits are considered to be alkaline producing foods. Anything with a PH greater than 7 is considered to be alkaline and is non-acidic. When it comes to foods, it is not the acid in the food that matters, but rather what occurs in your body once the food is consumed. For example, citrus fruit flesh and juice are acidic, but in your body they are alkaline-producing foods. Lemons, limes, avocados and kiwi are categorized as highly alkaline fruits and are therefore non-acidic. Other non-acidic fruits include bananas, cantaloupe, apples, coconut, grapefruit, grapes, oranges and watermelon.

Berries, which belong to the fruit group, are often found to be non-acidic and have an alkaline PH level. Strawberries, blackberries, black currants, raspberries and red currants are all non-acidic berries. Most berries will have a PH greater than 7. Exceptions are cranberries and blueberries, a couple of the few types of berries classified as acidic.

Non-Acidic Vegetables

The majority of vegetables contain an alkaline PH level and do not generate acids when consumed. You may need to be wary of some canned, frozen or pickled vegetables, however, since processing and packaging can change the PH level of these vegetables to become acidic. You don't need to worry about changes in PH level with fresh vegetables. Asparagus, broccoli, cucumbers, kale, beets, carrots, cabbage, Brussels sprouts, celery, lettuce, peppers, collard greens, pumpkin and onions are non-acidic vegetables.

Note that a food's acid or alkaline-forming tendency in the body has nothing to do with the actual PH of the food itself. For example, lemons are very acidic, however the end-products they produce after digestion and assimilation are alkaline so lemons are alkaline-forming in the body. Likewise, meat will test alkaline before digestion but it leaves acidic residue in the body so, like nearly all animal products, meat is classified as acid-forming.

It is important that your daily dietary intake of food naturally acts to balance your body PH. To maintain health, the diet should consist of at least 60% alkaline forming foods and at most 40% acid forming foods. To restore health, the diet should consist of 80% alkaline forming foods and 20% acid forming foods. The principles are clear: eat plenty of vegetables, some fruit daily, and don't eat too much of dairy products, grain products, and direct protein from eggs, meat and fish (as is typically the case in Western diet).

But remember... you don't have to cut out all acid-forming foods - some are necessary, typically 40% - otherwise you probably wouldn't get enough protein and variety of nutrients, yet alone make interesting meals that you enjoy. But you DO want to shift the overall balance of your diet over toward the alkaline, and away from the excessively acid-forming diet of a quick-food culture.

Similarly, be sure to include your share of the high alkaline-forming foods to balance those low-acid foods you eat for their overall nutritional value. And make alkaline choices, e.g. better to have brown rice than white rice, even though both are on the acid-forming side, because it moves you in the right PH direction - less acid - and also it is more healthy and nutritious in other respects.

Detoxify with Fruit & Vegetable Juices

All natural, raw, vegetable and fruit juices are alkaline-producing. (Fruit juices become more acid-producing when processed and especially when sweetened.)

The Science: Why are acidic lemons alkaline-producing?

The answer is simply that when we digest the food, it produces alkaline residue. That's why we classify it as an alkaline food. When we digest a food it is chemically oxidized ('burned') to form water, carbon dioxide and an inorganic compound. The alkaline or acidic nature of the inorganic compound formed determines whether the food is alkaline or acid-producing. If it contains more sodium, potassium or calcium, it's classed as an alkaline food. If it contains more sulphur, phosphate or chloride, it's classed as an acid food.

What difference does it make to have toxic blood? In order for the body to remain healthy and alive, your body keeps a delicate and precise balance of blood PH at 7.365, which is slightly alkaline. The body does whatever it has to in order to maintain this balance. The problem is that most people have incredibly acid lifestyles. Acid is produced in your body whenever you have stress, upset emotions and when the food you eat is acid-forming.

The typical diet is significantly acidic. So what happens to your body when you're over-acid? Your body will store excess acid in your fat cells (which is why so many people have such trouble losing weight).

IMPROVE YOUR HEALTH AND WEIGHT LOSS

Any time your health is at risk, your metabolism slows down until the problem is resolved. Most people don't realize that acid is causing their health issues, so they continue the habits that cause it in the first place. A lot of people treat their health issues with medication… but medication only makes it worse! If you PH remains off-balance too long, metabolic dysfunction can occur. Metabolic dysfunction exacerbates health issues and makes weight loss much more difficult than it should be. It's completely possible to balance your PH naturally, with foods.

If you want to achieve a certain measure of weight loss and keep it off for good, then it's important to put certain controls into play. Without an active plan to change your lifestyle, the goals you set forth just won't be attainable. For anyone trying to lose weight, regardless of the goal that is set, it always starts with food. As they say, you are what you eat. If you shovel unhealthy food into your mouth and live off of processed and refined goods that are loaded with calories, carbs and fat content then you're going to end up with all of that unnecessary garbage being stored as fat. In the end, you will become a walking example of what not to eat and how not to live. The good news for anyone that wants to lose weight is that the same is true for healthy foods and a certain measure of exercise. Most people don't understand how they woke up and suddenly found themselves overweight. They can't trace it to any measurable or quantifiable event because it's not something that happened overnight. It's something that has happened over the course of years as the result of abuse to the body. First things first, I'd recommend reducing your sugar, alcohol and coffee intake.

Sugar, alcohol and coffee have been proven to affect your PH balance. Just one coffee can drop your PH by as much as 4 points. Drinking lemon water can help improve your PH levels. A lot of people think lemons are acidic, but they're actually very alkalizing. Drinking at least 10, 8-oz. glasses of lemon-infused water can help balance your PH.

Why Can't You Lose Weight?

Too much acid in your body can cause weight gain, fatigue, pain, and a host of other health problems. However, it's easy to balance your body chemistry to get your weight and health back on track.

The PH scale which measures the level of acid or alkalinity. Don't worry you don't need to be a biochemist to balance your body's PH. The PH scale is like a tug-of-war in your body. On one side there is the acid team and on the other side is the alkaline team. The middle is neutral. Most of what we eat and our lifestyle choices tip the balance in favor of acidity. Meat, dairy products, sugary foods, soda, and many other foods are all extremely acidifying to the body.

If you look at the function of fat you will find that a moderate amount of fat is not the enemy, you actually need some body fat, in fact it may be saving your life. Body fat is essential for the normal healthy function of many of the body's systems, such as, organs, bone marrow, the nervous system, and muscles. It's also used as energy.

Body acidity and body fat are intricately linked in a way that is generally unknown to most people. Fat is one of the body's primary defenses used to protect your blood PH. PH is a measurement that determines the level of acidity or alkalinity. Your blood must maintain a PH of 7.3 to 7.4 to sustain life. And when your body's overall PH level is off there is low oxygen delivery to cells, creating an environment where disease thrives, setting the stage for many normally healthy processes to turn destructive.

41

To maintain proper PH levels, the body flushes out and removes as many acids and toxins as it can through sweating, urination, and defecation. When there are more toxins/acids than the body is able to dispose of, it produces toxic waste storage cells (fat cells) to store them in. So, you see, fat cells perform an important health function when they store toxins and excess acid. You may not appreciate the extra fat, but if you're PH is out of balance you may need these fat storage cells to sustain life.

This is an important concept to understand... If you are ingesting toxic chemical food ingredients, such as artificial sweeteners, monosodium glutimate (MSG), unhealthy oils, high fructose corn syrup, preservatives, or processed foods or exposing yourself regularly to other poisons and chemicals, like chemical based sunscreens, bug sprays, and body care products, as well as environmental toxins, then your body is working overtime to produce more and more fat cells to store these excessive toxins in.

That may be the answer to why dieting, exercise and discipline may not solve your weight issues. With respect to losing weight, you and your body may not have the same goal.

Genetics

There's no question that genes can play an important role in how you break down calories and store fat. But to blame your DNA for the more difficult challenge of losing weight wouldn't be right.

However, it is important to recognize that, except in very rare cases, the genes that impact body weight do not directly cause obesity. Rather, genetic makeup influences the susceptibility to weight gain when the person lives in an environment that supports eating calories in excess and/or limiting physical activity.

Obviously, everyone can't go for genetic testing before embarking on a weight loss effort. And where the rubber meets the road, it may not even matter what specific genetic makeup you have that could be adding to your difficulty.

Research shows - once again - that the calories-in, calories-out explanations about body weight are just too simplistic and don't account for many very real variables that have nothing to do with will or self-restraint. Many people have always known this at gut level, but it's good to see the science bear that out.

So if you're one of those with the bad hand, don't give up! A dietary and weight management program could be tailored to address your very specific needs in order to get and keep your weight in check. Because getting dealt a bad hand doesn't doom you to losing the game-it just means you need a different strategy for winning it.

It is not fully understood how this genetic factor works. It has something to do with the control of appetite. When you eat, certain hormones and brain chemicals send messages to parts of your brain to say that you have had enough and to stop eating. In some people, this control of appetite and the feeling of fullness (satiety) may be faulty, or not as good as it is in others.

How do I know if my weight is already affecting my health?

If you are worried that you are overweight or obese, you should discuss this with your doctor. They may be able to determine if your weight is already affecting your health.

For example, they may start by checking whether you have any symptoms of coronary heart disease such as chest pains, particularly on exertion. They may also ask about any symptoms of osteoarthritis such as back pain or joint pains, or any symptoms of sleep. This occurs when your breathing patterns are disturbed while you are sleeping, due to excess weight around your chest, neck and airways. They may suggest some tests to screen for any underlying health problems that may be caused by your weight.

How can I lose weight?

Some people lose weight by strict dieting for a short period. However, as soon as their diet is over, they often go back to their old eating habits and their weight goes straight back on. Losing weight and then keeping it off needs a change in your lifestyle for life.

This includes. The type of food and drink that you normally buy. The type of meals that you eat. Your pattern of eating. and The amount of physical activity that you do.

There's no rule that says that you should want to lose weight just because everyone else seems to be making that a priority in the new year. For some people, such as those who have a history of disordered eating, the basic strategies for weight loss (eating fewer calories, exercising more, or both) might not be a healthy choice, and they should check in with a doctor before making changes to their diet or workout habits. If you do want to start a weight-loss plan, it is important to keep a few things in mind.

 For one, setting your intentions and understanding your motivation for wanting to lose weight helps keep you focused on what you need and want out of the journey, so that you never lose sight of what matters most: your health and happiness. Plus, there's so much that goes into weight loss that we often don't think about.

How much sleep you get, your stress levels, and health issues such as medications and hormones all play important roles in losing and maintaining weight. There's a lot to consider and no quick fix or magic bullet to give you lasting, sustainable change.

If you're trying to lose weight, you need to operate off a calorie deficit. That means burning more calories than you consume. To do this, focus on changing both your diet and exercise habits—just paying attention on one or the other isn't going to give you the results you want. If you lose 15 pounds in 4 weeks because you did something drastic, you'll likely put it back on when you go back to your old habits. "In the end, healthy eating and exercise is really what works. We're all looking for magic pill, but if that worked everyone would be thin, no one would have weight problems. It's not that easy. If it's too easy and the weight's flying off, you're probably doing something that's not maintainable.

STAY FOCUSED ON YOUR ACTIONS, NOT YOUR PROGRESS

Too many people approach their health with an all or nothing attitude. Good health should stem from the aim for continuous healthy lifestyle choices. By making small, positive decisions every day, you will be on your way to a healthier you. Small things like drinking a glass of water instead of soft drink, or choosing salad instead of chips at dinner will move you closer to your goal. Use these daily positive actions as your benchmark for getting closer to your objectives.

Motivation is crucial

No weight loss plan will work unless you have a serious desire to lose weight. You need to be ready and motivated.

Set clear goals with a realistic timescale

it is important to set a clear and realistic weight loss goal. in most cases, health benefits can be gained from losing the first 5-10% of your weight.

Aim to eat a healthy balanced diet

Special diets which are often advertised are not usually helpful. This is because after losing weight, if your old eating habits remain, the weight often goes straight back on. It is usually not a special diet that is needed but changing to a healthy balanced diet, for good.

Meals Simple Delicious, healthy food doesn't have to contain a lot of ingredients. Keep your meal ingredients to a minimum—just be sure to include a source of whole grains, lean protein, and healthy fat at each meal. For example, veggies and shrimp stir fried in sesame oil over a bed of brown rice seems restaurant quality but can be whipped up faster than takeout.

Eat on a Regular Schedule

Try not to let more than about four hours go by between meals or snacks. Steady meal timing helps regulate your digestive system, blood sugar and insulin levels, and appetite.

Listen to Your Body

Eat when you're hungry and stop when you're full, meaning satisfied, not stuffed. The recipes here intentionally don't provide amounts. That's so you get used to relying on your hunger and fullness cues to tell you when to stop and start eating.

Eating Dinner

Lentils and Quinoa with Mint and Lemon: Sauté chopped red onion, minced garlic, celery, and red bell pepper in extra virgin olive oil until tender. Add lentils (vacuum sealed or canned, rinsed, and drained are both fine) to heat through. Serve over a small scoop of cooked quinoa and garnish with fresh mint and juice from a fresh lemon wedge.

Tuna Lettuce Wraps with Basil Pesto and Couscous: Fill large outer romaine lettuce leaves with a mixture of drained chunk light tuna canned in water tossed with basil pesto, minced sun-dried tomatoes and whole wheat couscous.

Avocado, Beans, and Lime: Mix mashed avocado with minced onion, tomato, fresh lime juice, and cilantro. Toss with torn romaine to coat leaves. Top with a small scoop each of frozen, thawed corn and black beans

Clean-Eating

Seared Shrimp in Coconut Oil: On the stovetop, sear fresh shrimp in coconut oil and season with fresh grated ginger and scallions. Serve over a bed of mixed field greens and top with fresh pear slices.

Spaghetti Squash with Garlic, Mushrooms, Tomato and, Feta: Sauté chopped onions, minced garlic, sliced mushrooms, and a small, diced plum tomato in extra virgin olive oil. Reduce to low heat to keep warm. Slice a small spaghetti squash in half, remove seeds, place face down in a glass dish with a few tablespoons of water. Cover with wax paper and microwave on high for 7 to 8 minutes. Rake out strands, toss with sautéed veggies, and garnish with crumbled feta cheese.

Clean-Eating

Pineapple Chicken with a Twist: Stir fry sliced red and green bell peppers and a dash of crushed red pepper in sesame oil. Add diced, cooked chicken breast and pineapple chunks to heat through. Serve over a scoop of cooked wild rice.

The foundation of all clean-eating plans is limiting (or eliminating) all packaged and processed foods. But some recommendations include elimination of red meat, gluten and dairy. Others espouse juicing to 'rest" your digestive tract (nothing could be further from the truth: food is the best workout for your digestive tract). Before you start any plan, always talk to your doctor before eliminating whole nutrient groups from your diet.

Clean eating is a concept that must be followed regularly, over time, to reap any health benefits. But you don't need to be a perfect eater —no one is! If you stick with these recommendations at least 80 percent of the time – give yourself a little "wiggle room" – you'll feel more satisfied after eating and boost your energy level.

The best — and easiest — clean-eating strategy would be quite familiar to our parents and grandparents. It's a "one-size-fits-all" eating plan supporting a healthy heart, brain, and digestive tract.

Avoid most packaged and processed foods

The first step in clean eating. Read labels to avoid added sugars, salts, and fats. While bagged, boxed, or canned foods can be a convenience - especially for healthy, out of season foods (think canned tomatoes), make the habit of looking for added sugars, salt, and fats. You can always "correct" the flavors if you choose, with your own additions.

Choose real foods Look for foods that you can recognize in their whole, natural state. Choose seasonal fruits and vegetables for optimal nutrient density and freshness. And include frozen fruits and vegetables in the mix (without sauces). You'll save money and enjoy out-out-season produce, like blueberries in winter.

Cut back on added sugars

All humans are born with a "sweet tooth". And fruit is nature's candy. Fresh or dried, before there was candy, cookies, cake and other vehicles for loads of added sugars, we turned to fruit. Portable, economical, and a treat for your taste buds. And there is a range of sweetness in fruits. Slightly under-ripe fruit is on the lower end of the sweetness scale, while super-ripe and dried fruits concentrate and boost the sweetness signals.

Avoid trans-fats/ Limit saturated fats

Swap out unhealthy, artery-clogging fats from all sources to healthy ones. Processed and packaged foods are the main sources of trans fats, but meat also contains small amounts. Saturated fats are found in fatty meats, full fat dairy, butter, and Use heart-healthy plant-based oils like nuts, olives, and avocado.

Cook and eat at home

While not a food-specific recommendation, when you cook at home you know the ingredients and seasonings in every dish. No guesswork or taste-testing for hidden fats, salt, and sugar found in restaurant meals and prepared foods. You can personalize your eating with spices and herbs instead of salt, smaller amounts of healthy fats, and a lot less sugar.

Stay hydrated Our bodies need abundant water for optimal function. And while fruits and vegetables are mostly water and contribute a large portion of daily fluid needs, added fluids are needed daily. While the newest guidelines suggest drinking "when thirsty", most people ignore these signals, or don't really recognize them. Aim for at least 6 glasses of water daily (which also includes non-caffeinated drinks, like herbal teas and coffee and seltzer). Spruce up your water with a slice of fruit, or even cucumber and mint.

Limit caffeine

New science fully documents the health benefits of moderate amounts of caffeine. Caffeine can boost alertness, energy, and mental focus when used modestly.

As caffeine intake rises, so do negative side effects including jitteriness, anxiety, stomach upset, and insomnia.

Aim for up to 300 mg daily, which is about 2 large mugs of coffee (typical coffeehouse size of 16 - 20 ounces), or 4 large mugs of tea.

If you find you're "caffeine-sensitive" with these guidelines, as many people are, cut back to an amount that is symptom-free for you.

Lose Weight Naturally

Foods that are packed with nutrients like fiber, vitamins, and minerals, will leave you feeling full and satisfied long after meals.

Glowing Health

There's an old saying that you are what you eat, and every bit of that is true.

What the body is fed directly impacts how the body looks and performs. When natural and clean foods are put into the body, improvements in skin, complexion, hair, nails, eyes, and waistline will follow. Adding greens to the diet will leave less room for junk food and increase energy levels and nourishment.

Start by eating greens at two meals per day. Add them as an appetizer or side dish. It does not matter if it's kale, spinach, or romaine lettuce, the point is to start making green appear on your plate, often.

Put lots of color on every plate.

The different colors signify the different vitamins and minerals that particular food.

Tomatoes get their bright red color from lycopene, which is a powerful cancer-fighting phytochemical, while carrots get their bright orange coat from the carotene, which is an antioxidant that plays a vital role in the health of the eyes.

Drink clean.

Not only is the majority of the world dehydrated, but they are also hydrated with the wrong things.

A big part of understanding the clean eating basics is knowing what to drink when unhealthy drinks are not an option.

Sugary drinks and diet sodas are full of artificial sweeteners and chemicals causing lasting damage to the body's stomach acids along with unwanted weight gain in the WORST PLACES. When it comes to fruits and vegetables, most of us aren't getting enough. Per the Centers for Disease Control and Prevention, 76 percent of Americans don't get enough fruit each day and a whopping 87 percent aren't eating enough servings of vegetables. Eating more fruit and vegetables can help significantly reduce your risk for a number of chronic diseases, including high blood pressure, type 2 diabetes, heart disease, obesity and cancer. The fiber in whole produce also helps keep your microbiome (the collection of good bacteria that live in your gut) happy, which can reduce your risk for autoimmune diseases, fight off pathogens and infections and even improve your mood.

Go Whole Grain

The cleanest whole grains are the ones that have been touched the least by processing. Think whole grains that look most like their just-harvested state—quinoa, wild rice, oats. While some people abstain from eating any processed grains, we think that whole-wheat pasta and whole-grain bread made with simple ingredients are part of eating clean. Sometimes you just need a hearty slice of avocado toast or a bowl of pasta. Don't get duped by "whole-grain" claims on labels though, to eat clean packaged whole grains you're going need to take a closer look at the ingredients. Whole grains should always be the first ingredient, the ingredient list should be short and recognizable, and it should have minimal (if any) added sugar. When you swap out refined carbs (like white pasta, sugar, and white bread) for whole grains you'll get more fiber, antioxidants and inflammation-fighting phytonutrients. Plus, people who eat more whole grains have an easier time losing weight and keeping it off long term.

Eat Less Meat

More and more research suggests cutting back on meat is healthier for you and the planet. Veganism isn't a requirement for clean eating though—just eating less meat can help reduce your blood pressure, reduce your risk of heart disease and help keep your weight in check. Plus, eating more plants helps bump up the fiber, healthy fats and vitamins and minerals in your diet. And if you're worried about getting enough protein by cutting down on meat— that shouldn't be an issue. Most Americans get much more than the recommended 0.8 grams of protein per kilogram of body weight (approximately 56 grams daily for men and 46 grams daily for women) and it's easy to get that much protein eating a vegetarian or even vegan diet. Eggs, dairy (with no added sugar and simple ingredients) When you do eat meat, choose options that haven't been pumped with antibiotics and even better if they've lived and eaten like they would in the wild (think grass-fed beef, wild-caught salmon). Clean eating also means cutting down on processed meats like cold cuts, bacon and sausage.

Limit Sugar

Most people eat too many added sugars. The American Heart Association recommends no more than about 6 teaspoons per day for women and 9 teaspoons per day for men. The average American gets about 4 times that amount—28 teaspoons of added sugar per day. To clean up your diet, cut down on added sugars by limiting sweets like soda, candy and baked goods. But it's more than just desserts—keep an eye on sugars added to healthier foods like yogurt (choose plain), tomato sauce and cereal. Look for foods without sugar as an ingredient, or make sure it's listed towards the bottom, which means less of it is used in the food. And you don't have to worry as much about naturally occurring sugars in fruit and dairy. They come packaged with fiber, protein or fat to help blunt the effect of sugar on insulin levels. They also deliver nutrients so you're not just getting empty, sugary calories.

Keep an Eye on Sodium

Just like with sugar, most of us are getting far more sodium than we should. The Institute of Medicine recommends capping sodium at 2,300 milligrams daily, about one teaspoon of salt. If you're over 50, of African-American descent or have high blood pressure, chronic kidney disease or diabetes, you may want to go even lower, to 1,500 milligrams per day. 80 percent of the sodium in our diets is coming from convenience foods. Cutting back on processed foods will help you reduce your salt intake, as most packaged foods contain more sodium than homemade versions. To help minimize salt while you cook, flavor your food with herbs and spices, citrus and vinegar. Clean eating recipes can still use salt, it is essential for bringing out the flavor of foods, but we use it smartly and sparingly. Coarse sea salt or kosher salt can add punch when sprinkled on dishes at the end of cooking, and they contain less sodium (teaspoon for teaspoon) compared to table salt.

Consider the Environment

Clean eating is better for you and the planet. The food we eat takes resources to get to our plate. According to some estimates, agriculture may account for one third of all greenhouse gas emissions. The meat industry is one of the biggest offenders. It takes a lot of resources to raise and feed an animal and the methane released from digestion and manure (especially for cows, goats and sheep) makes that carbon footprint even bigger. Some modern fishing practices have destroyed natural marine habitats and overfished certain species of seafood. Produce production can also take a toll with the types of herbicides, pesticides and synthetic fertilizers impacting water and soil quality. Eating clean comes in because going vege heavy and light on the meat can help preserve earth's resources. A vegetarian diet requires 3 times less water and 2.5 times less energy to produce than a meat-heavy diet. Broccoli has a carbon footprint that's 13 times lower than that of the same amount of conventionally raised beef. Shifting from a meat-forward style of eating to a plant-based style could slash greenhouse gas emissions—as well as add about a decade to your life, per a study in Nature. Choosing organic or grass-fed meat and purchasing sustainably-caught or farmed seafood makes your proteins a more environmentally-sound choice. Fruits and vegetables can be purchased organic, as well as local and in-season to help cut down on their carbon footprint.

Chapter 7

Best PH Health Benefits

The avocado is a rather unique type of fruit. Most fruit consists primarily of carbohydrate, while avocado is high in healthy fats. Numerous studies show that it has powerful beneficial effects on health. Avocados are a stone fruit with a creamy texture that grow in warm climates. Their potential health benefits include improving digestion, decreasing risk of depression, and protection against cancer.

Eating a diet that contains plenty of fruits and vegetables of all kinds has long been associated with a reduced risk of many lifestyle-related health conditions. Numerous studies have found that a predominantly plant-based diet that includes foods such as avocados can help to decrease the risk of obesity, diabetes, heart disease. Although most of the calories in an avocado come from fat, don't shy away! Avocados are full of healthy, beneficial fats that help to keep you full. When you consume fat, your brain receives a signal to turn off your appetite. Eating fat slows the breakdown of carbohydrates, which helps to keep sugar levels in the blood stable. Fat is essential for every single cell in the body. Eating healthy fats supports skin health, enhances the absorption of fat-soluble vitamins, minerals, and other nutrients, and may even help boost the immune system. Avocados have more potassium than sodium, which is good news for the heart since potassium lowers blood pressure, while sodium raises it. Every 100 g avocado has 485 mg potassium and 7 mg sodium. Potassium is also important for normal heart function as it aids skeletal and smooth muscle contraction. Having more potassium can actually help patients of high blood pressure and lower the risk of strokes by 24%.6 High cholesterol is a dangerous condition that raises your risk for several diseases, including heart attacks. But not all cholesterol is bad. While LDL cholesterol is harmful, HDL cholesterol is actually good for your health. It also helps remove the extra LDLs. People with high cholesterol also have a fat called triglycerides, too much of which is bad for you.

Avocado is delicious fruits are able to increase levels of "good" (HDL) cholesterol and lower levels of LDL cholesterol, making avocados a perfect addition to increase the strength and health of your cardiovascular system.

It is believed that avocados are soothing for the intestine and therefore aid on digestion. They contain soluble and insoluble fibers that help to keep the digestive system running smoothly. These types of fiber are very important for digestion because they bulk up stools and help ensure the smooth passage of food through the intestinal tract. Furthermore, they stimulate gastric and digestive juices so nutrients are absorbed in the most efficient and rapid way. Finally, they reduce the symptoms from conditions like constipation and diarrhea. All in all, the huge amount of fiber found in avocados (40% of daily requirement per serving) makes this a very important food for optimizing your digestive health.

Liver Care Avocados are very good at reducing liver damage. It has certain organic compounds that help in improving liver health. Liver damage is normally caused due to Hepatitis C. Findings of a recent research study suggest that avocados may play a major role in toning up and protecting your liver from a wide variety of conditions.

Improves Vision

Avocados help keep your eyes healthy. They contain carotenoids such as lutein and zeaxanthin, which help to protect your eyes against cataracts, eye diseases related to age, and macular degeneration. These conditions are often caused by free radicals that accumulate in the tissues of the eyes. The antioxidant activity of these special carotenoids in avocados neutralize the effects of those dangerous free radicals.

Promotes Healthy Heart

The health benefits of avocados include a healthier heart. Beta-sitosterol, which is found in avocados, helps maintain healthy cholesterol levels. Research studies suggest that the intake of avocado may enhance antiatherogenic properties of HDL cholesterol, which helps in protecting the heart from atherosclerosis, also known as arteriosclerotic vascular disease. The significant levels of potassium also make avocados a powerful fruit in the fight against hypertension. Potassium is a vasodilator, which relaxes the tension of blood vessels and arteries, thereby reducing the chances of clotting, heart attacks, and strokes.

Anti-cancer Properties Health benefits of avocados include a lower risk of cancers, including breast cancer and prostate cancer. Avocado contains carotenoids and monounsaturated fat, both of which contribute to the significant reduction of cancer. Avocado also contains Glutathione, an antioxidant that protects the cells from cancer and the dangerous effects of free radicals. The list of antioxidant and anti-inflammatory compounds in avocados is impressive, and it is almost difficult to determine which one has the largest impact. Studies have been widely done on oral, skin, and prostate cancers, and the results show that instead of metastasizing, the organic compounds in avocados cause cancerous cells to undergo apoptosis (automatic cell death). Research is still ongoing on the relationship between avocados and cancer.

Avocado is alkaline

 You heard that correct You might have heard about "The alkaline diet", which basically encourages people to eat more alkaline forming foods. If you paid attention in chemistry class than you might know that there are acids and bases, which are measured in PH. Solutions with a pH less than 7 are acidic, solutions with a PH greater than 7 are basic or alkaline.

Avocados have an unusual and brilliant fat profile

During the low fat dynasty avocados got a bad reputation because 85% of their calories come from fat. But we know better now: the type of fat matters. Healthy fats are essential to a healthy body and avocados got them.

Avocados are rich in monounsaturated fat, which is easily burned for energy. Monounsaturated fat might also help to decrease total cholesterol levels, which lowers the risk of heart disease. They also help to regulate blood sugar, which is great news for everyone not only for those who struggle with diabetes or weight gain. One avocado delivers about 40% of your daily needs for fiber. This is positive in many ways. Fiber helps lower cholesterol levels Fiber also maintains a steady blood sugar level because it slows down the breakdown of carbohydrates. This will make you feel full for longer, which aids in achieving a healthy weight.

Avocados contain glutathione

The body produces glutathione but medications, stress and poor diet can deplete glutathione levels. A deficiency in glutathione has been linked to disease like diabetes, arthritis, heart disease, dementia and Alzheimer disease. Eating avocados therefore is a natural way to boost glutathione levels.

Avocados have an fantastic carotenoid diversity

In addition to supplying folate, copper, potassium, vitamin K, C, D and B6, avocados provide a kingdom of carotenoids (like lutein, beta-carotene, alpha-carotene). Carotenoids are the organic pigments that are found in plants and other organisms. They are powerful antioxidants that can help prevent disease like cancer and enhance your immune response to infections. It's been said that if you add avocado to your salad the absorption of carotenoids is increased between 200-400%. That alone is a reason to enjoy more of this green super fruit.

Avocados are most beneficial when they are ripe . Over-ripe avocados will be darker in color, almost a dark brown or black color. When you peel a just right avocado it should be a nice bright green color. If there are any dark brown spots when peeled, it is too ripe. It is best to buy the avocados un-ripen and you can allow them to ripen in your home at room temperature. To make them ripen faster you can store them in a bag with apples or bananas. To slow down the process of ripening you can store the avocado in your refrigerator.

Garlic Nutritional Values

Garlic is a plant from the same family as onion. Traditionally used as flavoring for food, in the last years garlic has also been used as a medicine to prevent and treat a wide range of diseases and conditions. Fresh or cooked cloves are used for consumption, while both supplements and cloves are used for medicinal purposes.

It is generally accepted that garlic has important applications in medicine, but there are still debates regarding its effectiveness on some particular conditions. Each person is different and unless garlic poses a safety concern such as allergy, eating it regularly will be like eating any other food.

Lowers blood pressure and cholesterol

Reduces risk of coronary diseases, heart attack, atherosclerosis Prevents cold, flu and fever Prevents and ameliorates enlarged prostate Maintains healthy liver functions Prevents cancer Lowers blood levels Fights bacterial and fungal infections.

Garlic in Alkaline Diet

Garlic is a good source of nutrients and can also be used as medicine. Being highly alkaline, it helps regulating body pH so it is a valuable addition to the diet. Used raw, it adds spice to the foods and maintains the whole range of nutrients. Some supplements are odorless but this only means that allicin, which is the main ingredient, is less or old, thus the effectiveness of the product is lower.

Eat more Garlic

In order to help strengthening your immune system, eat a raw clove every day.

Whatever activity you decide to choose, garlic will make it last longer. Before you start to eat garlic you can probably manage just 30 minutes of exercise and it would be hard to imagine the effects that would have on your body. After eating garlic, you will definitely last over an hour and you can even do a lot more exercise like cardio exercises then lifting weights after that. One more health benefit of eating garlic is that it improves bone health which means it has a lot of vitamins in it. It is definitely healthy than most people think so include it in your grocery list.

One of the most popular benefits of garlic is that it lowers the risk of heart disease. There is no doubt one of the leading causes of death in the world is heart attack which could cause you to drop dead no matter where you are. If there is nobody near you to get you to the nearest hospital then your chances for survival are slim to none. The best way to prevent this type of disease is to eat garlic and you don't have to eat garlic only. You can eat it while it is mixed with your favorite food. Besides, a lot of food become even more delicious when mixed with garlic and some chefs have admitted that fact.

One benefit it has is that it reduces cold which is good news for those who always gets a rough case of colds. It is a common disease and it can even be transferable from one person to another. It is better to treat it naturally instead of relying on medicine because you can get immune to medicine. Whether you decide to purchase red garlic or white garlic it is still equally good for your health.

Eat an Alkaline Diet

If there's such thing as a pH balance diet, it's one that includes lots of green plants and other alkalizing foods. It's also smart to purchase as much organic food as possible, since crops that are grown in organic, mineral-dense soil tend to be more alkalizing and have higher vitamin and mineral content. Here are foods that are included in a well-rounded alkaline diet:

Leafy green vegetables — for example, kale, chard, beet greens, dandelion, spinach, wheat grass, alfalfa grass, etc. Other non-starchy veggies — including mushrooms, tomatoes, avocado, radishes, cucumber, broccoli, oregano, garlic, ginger, green beans, endive, cabbage, celery, zucchini and asparagus.

Raw foods — Uncooked fruits and vegetables are said to be biogenic or "life-giving." Cooking foods depletes alkalinizing minerals. Increase your intake of raw foods, and try juicing or lightly steaming fruits and vegetables. Ideally try to consume a good portion of your produce raw or only lightly cooked (such as steamed), as raw foods can help supply high levels of alkalizing minerals.

Healthy fats — these include coconut oil, MCT oil or virgin olive oil (fats found in wild-caught fish, grass-fed beef, cage-free eggs, nuts, seeds and organic grass-fed butter are also good additions to your diet, even if they aren't necessarily alkalizing).

Most fruits — Strangely enough, acidic fruits such as grapefruit and tomatoes don't create acidity in the body. They do just the opposite and contribute to an alkaline environment. Citrus fruits, dates and raisins are all very alkalizing and may help prevent acidosis.

Most fruits — Strangely enough, acidic fruits such as grapefruit and tomatoes don't create acidity in the body. They do just the opposite and contribute to an alkaline environment. Citrus fruits, dates and raisins are all very alkalizing and may help prevent acidosis.

Baking Soda

Baking soda is highly alkaline and can assist in balancing your body's pH, Drink a large 8 oz. glass of water mixed with 1/2 tsp. baking soda several times a day for a quick adjustment in pH levels, Baking soda can raise your blood pressure, so if you take medicines for hypertension or have untreated high blood pressure, avoid consuming baking soda unless you are under medical supervision. not drinking more than a total of 4 tsp. baking soda daily, but to only consume this amount if you are seriously ill. Consult your health practitioner for dosing directions.

Alkaline Foods

Eat foods that are naturally alkaline, suggests "The PH Miracle." Foods like parsley and alfalfa sprouts have a high pH making them very alkaline in their raw form. Add them to salads and as garnishes to your meals or make freshly squeeze vegetables juices including these foods. Other highly alkaline foods are all melons, figs, watermelon, most ripe fruits, asparagus, kelp, other seaweeds, watercress, wheatgrass and most herbal teas. It is always better to eat these foods in their raw state to obtain their highest nutritional values.

Fruit Juices

Most fruit is alkaline-forming and will raise the body's pH levels. Even citrus fruits become alkaline during the digestive process. Good choices for fruits to juice for a more alkaline system are apples, ripe bananas, grapes, peaches, nectarines, pears, mangos, oranges, grapefruit, pineapples, pomegranate and berries of all kinds. Several fruits are slightly acidic, including cranberries, prunes and plums, and should be consumed in moderation if your goal is to raise pH levels.

Green Smoothies

Green smoothies can provide the best of both fruits and vegetables in a drink that is filling enough to serve as a meal replacement. Blends of kale, spinach and sprouts with melon, kiwi, orange juice or strawberries are loaded with vitamins and antioxidants and are alkaline. Apple juice, celery, spinach and grapes are equally well-balanced. Ripe banana thickens blended juice to shake consistency and adds sweetness to a smoothie.

Vegetable Juices

Alkaline vegetables you can toss into a juicer or blender include celery, broccoli, leaf lettuces and greens of all kinds. Carrot juice is alkaline-forming and combines well with other alkaline fruits and vegetables for a sweet, nutritious drink. Try carrot and celery or carrot and apple juice for something simple to raise PH. Tomatoes are tasty when juiced with herbs, garlic, celery, cabbage, parsley and other veggies. The highest nutrition comes from juice you make and drink fresh, but you can use a commercial low-sodium, organic vegetable juice as an occasional alternative.

Acidosis

In a constant state of acidosis, your body uses its available minerals to help balance its pH levels. Calcium is the most important mineral your body uses to neutralize acid. When your body repeatedly leaches calcium from your bones, you may start to develop conditions such as osteoporosis. Acidosis is also a major factor in stressing your body and increasing your Cortisol levels, which affects sleep patterns. Acidosis can cause kidney stones, lower growth hormones, increased body fat and a reduction in muscle mass.

Risk of an Imbalance

Your body constantly works to maintain a proper pH balance between 7.35 and 7.45. As a reference, the pH of pure water is 7. When your pH levels fall below 7.35, clinically you have acidosis and your central nervous system will start to depress. If your pH level falls below 7, you have severe acidosis, which can cause a coma and ultimately become fatal. When your pH level rises above 7.45, you have alkalosis. Alkalosis makes your nervous system hypersensitive, resulting in muscle spasms and convulsions.

Foods That Form Acids

Some foods are more acidic than others. By avoiding overly acidic foods, you can help balance the pH levels in your body. Dairy products, including all types of cheeses, butter and milk, are acidic. Meat from venison, wild game, poultry, shellfish, coldwater fish and cattle is also acidic. Other acidic products include many prescription drugs, coffee, soft drinks, alcohol, soy and whey protein isolates, margarine and synthetic.

All vegetables are alkalizing. If you simply eat more vegetables, you're well on your way to a more alkaline diet. It's best to eat Raw or steamed is excellent. All types of seaweed are particularly alkalizing. Greens, such as spinach, parsley, kale and watercress are also highly rated. This includes herbal teas and fresh vegetable juices.

Don't forget to add Chia seed to your diet

Chia Seeds Are High in Quality Protein Chia seeds contain a decent amount of protein. By weight, they are about 14 percent protein, which is very high compared to most plants. They also contain a good balance of essential amino acids, so our bodies should be able to make use of the protein in them. Protein has all sorts of benefits for health. It is also the most weight loss friendly nutrient in the diet, by far. A high protein intake reduces appetite and has been shown to reduce obsessive thoughts about food by 60 percent percent and the desire for night time snacking by 50 percent. Chia seeds really are an excellent protein source, especially for people who eat little or no animal products. Bottom Line: Chia seeds are high in quality protein, much higher than most plant foods. Protein is the most weight loss friendly macronutrient and can drastically reduce appetite and cravings. Like flax seeds, chia seeds are very high in Omega-3 fatty acids. In fact, chia seeds contain more Omega-3s than salmon, gram for gram. Chia Seeds May Improve Certain Blood Markers, Which Should Lower The Risk of Heart Disease and Type 2 Diabetes. Given that chia seeds are high in fiber, protein and Omega-3s, they should be able to improve metabolic health. This has been tested in several studies.

Chia Seeds Can Cause Major Improvements in Type 2 Diabetics

The most successful application of chia seeds to date was in a study on type 2 diabetic patients. In this study, 20 diabetic patients received either 37 grams of chia seeds, or 37 grams of wheat bran, for 12 weeks. When they got the chia seeds, they saw improvements in several important health markers. Given that chia seeds are high in fiber, it does seem plausible that they could help reduce blood sugar spikes after meals.

Chia Seeds In Your Diet

The seeds themselves taste rather bland, so you can add them to pretty much anything. which makes them much easier to prepare. They can be eaten raw, soaked in juice, added to porridges and puddings or added to baked goods. You can also sprinkle them on top of cereal, yogurt, vegetables or rice dishes. Because of their ability to absorb both water and fat, they can be used to thicken sauces. They can also be mixed with water and turned into a gel. Adding chia seeds to recipes will dramatically boost the nutritional value.

Beets

Beets and other vegetables tend to be richer in minerals, and they're also one of the best foods for helping to raise pH levels. Plus, it offers a wealth of other health benefits too, as one of the few sources of a phytonutrient known as betalain, which is believed to offer cancer prevention properties.

Sea vegetables

Sea vegetables like kelp, dulse, nori, and wakame are excellent alkaline foods as some of the most mineral-rich foods on Earth, packed with potassium and magnesium as well as vitamin A, C and K. You can use sea veggies by adding them to a soup or salad, and, if you're avoiding gluten or grains, you can use Nori wraps as a substitute for a grain-based wrap.

Hemp seeds

Hemp has often been classified as one of nature's most perfect foods, and it's probably no surprise that it's considered to be an alkaline food as well. That's because it's loaded with chlorophyll, which is known to be alkalizing, helping to combat acidity while normalizing the body's pH, as well as aiding in cleansing, healing, and detoxification. These tiny seeds are also powerhouses of dietary fiber, antioxidants, vitamins and minerals, like calcium, vitamin D, vitamin B, vitamin E, iron, magnesium, zinc, copper, manganese, and phosphorus. Add hemp seeds to a smoothie, yogurt, oatmeal, salad, or simply snack on them alone. To enjoy the benefits, just be sure that they are 100% raw and organic.

Spirulina Spirulina is a form of sea algae, but it's not a sea vegetable. This super food is hard to beat when it comes to alkalizing the blood, and on top of that, it contains 80 percent of the daily recommended value for iron, most of your requirements for B vitamins, and, it's loaded with vitamin A – containing more than 800 percent of your daily needs. Spirulina is also one of the few foods with a natural GLA content. Gamma Linolenic Acid. GLA is difficult to find in a food source, and typically has to be created by the body. It offers anti-inflammatory properties and has been found to help combat chronic inflammation, eczema, dermatitis, asthma, rheumatoid arthritis, atherosclerosis, diabetes, obesity and even cancer.

Garlic

One of the most powerful superfoods of all, garlic is often at the top of foods lists for improving overall health, and it's also a top alkaline-forming food. Being highly alkaline, it helps regulate pH, but it also offers a host of other benefits, including lowering blood pressure and cholesterol, helping to prevent the flu or a cold, reducing the risk of heart disease, preventing cancer and fighting off fungal and bacterial infections. Garlic can add flavor and medicinal benefits to all sorts of dishes, like pasta sauce, salsas, homemade salad dressings and more. To maximize its benefits, before consuming or adding to a dish, chop it up and let it to rest for about 10 minutes. This allows its beneficial, health-promoting allicin content to form. For those with high cholesterol, garlic supplementation appears to reduce total and/or LDL cholesterol by about 12-15% Garlic contains antioxidants that support the body's protective mechanisms against oxidative damage.

Garlic May Help You Live Longer The combined effects on reducing cholesterol and blood pressure, as well as the antioxidant properties, may help prevent common brain diseases like Alzheimer's disease and dementia. Eating Garlic Can Help Detoxify Heavy Metals in the Body. At high doses, the sulfur compounds in garlic have been shown to protect against organ damage from heavy metal toxicity. Effects on longevity are basically impossible to prove in humans. But given the beneficial effects on important risk factors like blood pressure, it makes sense that garlic could help you live longer.

The fact that it can fight infectious disease is also an important factor, because these are common causes of death, especially in the elderly or people with dysfunctional immune systems. Garlic is an incredibly tasty herb linked to various health benefits. About 11% of garlic's fiber content comes from inulin and 6% from a sweet, naturally occurring prebiotic called fructooligosaccharides (FOS).

Garlic acts as a prebiotic by promoting the growth of beneficial Bifidobacteria in the gut. It also prevents disease-promoting bacteria from growing. Garlic extract may be effective for reducing the risk of heart disease, and has shown antioxidant, anti-cancer and antimicrobial effects. It may also have benefits against asthma. Garlic gives great flavor to your foods and provides you with prebiotic benefits. It has been shown to help promote good bacteria and prevent harmful bacteria from growing.

Onions Onions are a very tasty and versatile vegetable linked to various health benefits. Similar to garlic, inulin accounts for 10% of the total fiber content of onions, while FOS makes up around 6%

FOS strengthens gut flora, helps with fat breakdown and boosts the immune system by increasing nitric oxide production in cells. Onions are also rich in the flavonoid quercetin, which gives onions antioxidant and anticancer properties. Furthermore, onions have antibiotic properties and may provide benefits for the cardiovascular system. Onions are loaded with numerous health benefits, and scientists are still discovering how beneficial this vegetable really is. They're a very good source of vitamin C and B6, iron, folate, and potassium. The manganese content in onions provides cold and flu relief with its anti-inflammatory abilities.

Two phytochemical (plant-derived nutrient) compounds in onions – allium and allyl disulphide – convert to allicin when the bulb is cut or crushed due to enzyme activation. Studies show these compounds to have cancer- and diabetes-fighting properties, while decreasing blood vessel stiffness by releasing nitric oxide. This can reduce blood pressure, inhibit platelet clot formation, and help decrease the risk of coronary artery disease, peripheral vascular diseases, and stroke.

Significant amounts of polyphenols (another phytochemical in onions) and an antioxidant flavonoid called quercetin (which has proven anti-cancer, anti-inflammatory, and anti-diabetic functions) account for the reputation onions have for disease prevention.

Luckily, cooking onions in soup doesn't diminish their quercetin value – it simply transfers to the broth. The flavonoids in onions are more concentrated in the outer layers, so discard as little as possible.

Studies showed strong evidence that eating onions may considerably reduce the risk of stomach cancer

Since the dawn of time, onions have been used to liven up food recipes and added to ancient concoctions for medicinal purposes. Modern medicine has found onions to be highly beneficial in almost every area of the body, from maintaining cell health to preventing inflammation to purifying the blood. Onions also providing a savory goodness that blends well with other foods.

Asparagus

Asparagus is a popular vegetable and another great source of prebiotics. The inulin content may be around 2-3 grams per 100-gram (3.5-oz) serving. Asparagus has been shown to promote friendly bacteria in the gut and has been linked to the prevention of certain cancers The combination of fiber and antioxidants in asparagus also appears to provide anti-inflammatory benefits.

A 100-gram (3.5-oz) serving of asparagus also contains about 2 grams of protein.

Asparagus is a spring vegetable rich in prebiotic fiber and antioxidants. It promotes healthy gut bacteria and may help prevent certain cancers.

Bananas

Bananas are very popular. They're rich in vitamins, minerals and fiber. Bananas contain small amounts of inulin. Unripe (green) bananas are also high in resistant starch, which has prebiotic effects.

The prebiotic fiber in bananas has been shown to increase healthy gut bacteria and reduce bloating.

Oats

Whole oats are a very healthy grain with prebiotic benefits. They contain large amounts of beta-glucan fiber, as well as some resistant starch. Beta-glucan from oats has been linked to healthy gut bacteria, lower LDL cholesterol, better blood sugar. Whole oats are a grain rich in beta-glucan fiber. They increase healthy gut bacteria, improve blood sugar control and may reduce cancer risk.

Apples

Apples are a delicious fruit. Pectin accounts for approximately 50% of an apple's total fiber content. The pectin in apples has prebiotic benefits. It increases butyrate, a short-chain fatty acid that feeds the beneficial gut bacteria and decreases the population of harmful bacteria. Apples are also high in polyphenol antioxidants.

Apples are rich in pectin fiber. Pectin promotes healthy gut bacteria and helps decrease harmful bacteria. It also helps lower cholesterol.

Konjac Root

Konjac root, also known as elephant yam, is a tuber often used as a dietary supplement for its health benefits. Konjac glucomannan promotes the growth of friendly bacteria in the colon, relieves constipation and boosts your immune system.

The glucomannan fiber found in konjac root helps promote friendly bacteria, reduces constipation, boosts the immune system, lowers cholesterol in the blood and helps with weight loss.

Flaxseeds

Flaxseeds are incredibly healthy. They're also a great source of prebiotics. The fiber content of flaxseeds is 20–40% soluble fiber from mucilage gums and 60–80% insoluble fiber from cellulose and lignin. The fiber in flaxseeds promotes healthy gut bacteria, promotes regular bowel movements and reduces the amount of dietary fat you digest and absorb.

Because of their content of phenolic antioxidants, flaxseeds also have anti-cancer and antioxidant properties and help regulate blood sugar levels.

Yacon Root

Yacon root is very similar to sweet potatoes and is rich in fiber. It is particularly rich in prebiotic fructooligosaccharides (FOS) and inulin. The inulin in yacon has been shown to improve gut bacteria, reduce constipation, enhance the immune system, improve mineral absorption and regulate blood fats. Yacon root is rich in inulin and FOS.

It is great at promoting digestive health, improving mineral absorption, enhancing your immune system and regulating blood fats.

Seaweed

Seaweed (marine algae) is rarely eaten. However, it is a very potent prebiotic food. Approximately 50–85% of seaweed's fiber content comes from water-soluble fiber. Seaweed is also rich in antioxidants that have been linked to the prevention of heart attacks and strokes.

Seaweed is a great source of prebiotic fiber. It can increase the population of friendly bacteria, block the growth of harmful bacteria and enhance immune function.

Prebiotics Are Very Important

Prebiotic foods are high in special types of fiber that support digestive health. They promote the increase of friendly bacteria in the gut, help with various digestive problems and even boost your immune system. Prebiotic foods have also been shown to improve metabolic health and even help prevent certain diseases. However, some of the fiber content of these foods may be altered during cooking, so try to consume them raw rather than cooked. Do yourself and your gut bacteria a favor by eating plenty of these prebiotic foods.

Cayenne pepper As part of a family of potent peppers that contain enzymes essential to endocrine function, cayenne is considered to be one of the most alkalizing foods. It's known for its antibacterial properties as well as being an excellent source of vitamin A, helping to fight off harmful free radicals that lead to stress and disease. An added bonus? Eating cayenne peppers is also believed to help speed up the metabolism, promoting weight loss.

Lemons

While you might think that lemons are acidic, they're actually one of the most alkaline forming foods there is. This sour fruit provides powerful and immediate relief for hyperacidity and virus-related conditions, as well as coughs, colds, flu and heartburn too. Adding a squeeze of lemon to your water is a great way to add flavor to help ensure you're getting at least eight glasses of day, and drinking a glass of lemon water first thing in the morning is a great way to begin your day by getting those pH levels balanced out.

Celery

Celery is an outstanding alkalizing food. It's filled with vitamin C, vitamin K, natural electrolytes and lots of water, all important for helping to restore the body's balance, and preventing the loss of electrolytes which can lead to excess inflammation. It also contains a lesser-known nutrient, phthalides, which have been shown to lower cholesterol, as well as coumarin, known to inhibit a number of different cancers. Munching on celery is also known to help reduce high blood pressure, further reducing the risk of heart disease.

Broccoli

Broccoli is one of those vegetables that offers so much nutritional value and so many benefits that it is a must to include in your diet for better health. It's been proven time and again to be amazingly powerful for supporting the digestive and cardiovascular systems, inhibiting cancers, supporting the skin, immune system and metabolism. Eating it steamed or raw makes it an even more alkaline, nutritious food.

In addition to using broccoli in a stir-fry, you can steam it with other vegetables, use it in juices or smoothies, add it to a salad or eat it raw on its own.

Avocado

Avocado is a powerful, alkaline, nutrient-dense superfood. It contains healthy fats that can help prevent hunger pangs in between meals by keeping you feeling fuller and satisfied longer, and, thanks to its high content of oleic acid, it can help to lower total cholesterol, while raising levels of "good" or HDL cholesterol, and reducing "bad," or LDL cholesterol. Oleic acid also works to slow the development of heart disease and even speed up the metabolism to support weight loss. It also offers a host of other nutrients that offer anti-cancer, anti-inflammatory and blood sugar benefits.

Bell peppers

Bell peppers offer antioxidant superpower, are sweet, crunchy and can be used in almost any meal raw, roasted or grilled. This highly alkaline food contains flavonoids, carotenoids and hydroxycinnamic acids. In fact, bell peppers contain more than 30 different members of the carotenoid nutrient family – the only other food that comes close is the tomato. Bell peppers have been linked to a lower risk of cancer, inflammation, diabetes, cardiovascular disease and more.

Cucumber

This alkalizing food is 95% water. That makes it an astonishingly hydrating food, and cucumbers are also loaded with an incredible amount of antioxidants, including lignans, which have a significantly strong, scientifically proven reduced risk of cardiovascular disease and cancer, including ovarian, uterine, breast and prostate cancers.

Antioxidant Properties

Cucumbers contain numerous antioxidants, including the well-known vitamin C and beta-carotene. They also contain antioxidant flavonoids, such as quercetin, apigenin, luteolin, and kaempferol, 6 which provide additional benefits.

Freshen Your Breath

Placing a cucumber slice on the roof of your mouth may help to rid your mouth of odor-causing bacteria. According to the principles of Ayurveda, eating cucumbers may also help to release excess heat in your stomach, which is said to be a primary cause of bad breath.

Maintain a Healthy Weight

Cucumbers are very low in calories, yet they make a filling snack (one cup of sliced cucumber contains just 16 calories).8 The soluble fiber in cucumbers dissolves into a gel-like texture in your gut, helping to slow down your digestion. This helps you to feel full longer and is one reason why fiber-rich foods may help with weight control.**Cantaloupe**

This highly alkaline-forming, low-oxalate, nutrient-dense fruit contains 90 percent of the recommended daily allowance of vitamin C and 129 percent of the recommended daily allowance of vitamin B6. It's also an outstanding source of carotenes and potassium.

Cantaloupe is a delicious fruit having a variety of health benefits, including healthy skin and eyes, reduced chances of cancer, healthy lungs, and decreased stress levels. It also strengthens the immune system, prevents arthritis, and aids in managing diabetes. These attributes are mainly due to the high levels of vitamins and minerals that are present in this popular melon.

Cantaloupe Nutrition Facts

Cantaloupe is rich in many nutrients that provide various health benefits. It contains carbohydrates, protein, and water. Vitamins in a cantaloupe include vitamin A, beta-carotene, vitamin B1, vitamin B2, vitamin B6, vitamin B9, vitamin C, and vitamin K. The mineral wealth of this fruit includes potassium, calcium, iron, magnesium, phosphorus, and zinc.

Improves Vision

Vitamin C, zeaxanthin, and carotenoids present in cantaloupes are beneficial for maintaining healthy eyes. They are associated with a reduced risk of cataracts and macular degeneration.

Prevents Asthma

Cantaloupe is a rich source of vitamin C and beta-carotene. These nutrients are very helpful in lowering the risk of asthma.

Prevents Cancer

Cantaloupe aids in the prevention of cancer and the eradication of free radicals, the harmful by-products of cell metabolism that lead to a number of dangerous conditions. Cantaloupe is a rich source of beta-carotene, an essential carotenoid that the body requires. It works as an antioxidant and lowers the risk of different types of cancers, and the phytochemicals present in fresh fruits like cantaloupes have also been linked to anti-tumor behavior.

Skin & Hair Care

Cantaloupes contain dietary beta-carotene that ensures no overdose or vitamin A toxicity because the body only converts as much as it needs, unlike supplements; the rest remains as beta-carotene to fight diseases as antioxidants. The amount that turns into vitamin A enters the skin and stimulates the membrane of skin cells and increases growth and repair. This protects the skin membrane against harmful toxins that prematurely age the skin. Vitamin A cream is also used as a salve for irritation and redness on the skin, due to its naturally soothing qualities. Vitamin A is also good for sebum production, which helps keep the hair healthy and moisturized.

Boosts Immunity

Cantaloupe provides vitamin C, vitamin A, beta-carotene, and phytochemicals that work against free radicals. Vitamin C scavenges disease-causing free radicals and acts as an important line of defense for a healthy immune system. It also stimulates the production of white blood cells, which seek out and destroy dangerous bacteria, viruses, and other toxic substances or foreign bodies that may have found their way into our bloodstream.

Treats Arthritis

The phytochemicals in cantaloupes have anti-inflammatory qualities. This means that having a cantaloupe in your diet can help prevent oxidative stress on your joints and bones, thereby reducing inflammation. Chronic inflammation of these vital areas can lead to conditions like arthritis, so make sure to add plenty of cantaloupes to your diet if you're feeling creaky around the joints!

Controls Diabetes

Early research shows that cantaloupe is connected with improved insulin metabolism, which means a more stable fluctuation of blood sugar, preventing the dangerous spikes and plunges of blood sugar that all diabetics fear. It has also been shown to reduce oxidative stress on kidneys, which can further prevent a number of kidney-related diseases.

Kale Kale may be a trendy superfood these days, but with good reason. It's considered to be one of the most alkaline foods and is also widely known for its ability to aid the body in detoxification, lower total cholesterol and fight cancer. Similar to spinach, it has an astoundingly high amount of vitamin K, as well as vitamins C and A, in addition to its chlorophyll content, which as mentioned, is well-known to be alkalizing, helping to combat acidity while normalizing the body's pH, as well as aiding in cleansing, healing and detoxification.

One cup of kale has only 36 calories, 5 grams of fiber and 0 grams of fat. It is great for aiding in digestion and elimination with its great fiber content. It's also filled with so many nutrients, vitamins, folate and magnesium as well as those listed below.

Kale is high in iron.

Per calorie, kale has more iron than beef. Iron is essential for good health, such as the formation of hemoglobin and enzymes, transporting oxygen to various parts of the body, cell growth, proper liver function and more.

Kale is high in Vitamin K.

Eating a diet high in Vitamin K can help protect against various cancers. It is also necessary for a wide variety of bodily functions including normal bone health and blood clotting. Also increased levels of vitamin K can help people suffering from Alzheimer's disease. Kale has Antioxidants, such as carotenoids and flavonoids help protect against various cancers. Eating more kale can help lower cholesterol levels. Vitamin A is great for your vision, your skin as well as helping to prevent lung and oral cavity cancers. Kale is very helpful for your immune system, your metabolism and your hydration. kale has more calcium than milk, which aids in preventing bone loss, preventing osteoporosis and maintaining a healthy metabolism. Vitamin C is also helpful to maintain cartilage and joint flexibility. Kale is filled with fiber and sulfur, both great for detoxifying your body and keeping your liver healthy.

Detoxification and Weight loss

The fiber (5 grams in one cup) and sulfur in kale aid with digestion and liver health. The Vitamin C it contains hydrates your body and increases your metabolism, leading to weight loss and healthy blood sugar levels. The fiber in kale also lowers cholesterol.

Spinach

All leafy greens are important to include on an alkaline diet, and spinach is a favorite as it's so simple to use, extremely versatile and a nutritional powerhouse that's one of the top alkaline foods. As with all green veggies, it's rich in chlorophyll too. Spinach is also packed with vitamins K and A, folate, iron, manganese, magnesium, fiber.

Health Benefits of Spinach

Low in fat and even lower in cholesterol, spinach is high in niacin and zinc, as well as protein, fiber, vitamins A, C, E and K, thiamin, vitamin B6, folate, calcium, iron, magnesium, phosphorus, potassium, copper, and manganese. In other word, it's loaded with good things for every part of your body! Abundant flavonoids in spinach act as antioxidants to keep cholesterol from oxidizing and protect your body from free radicals, particularly in the colon. The folate in spinach is good for your healthy cardiovascular system, and magnesium helps lower high blood pressure. Studies also have shown that spinach helps maintain your vigorous brain function, memory and mental clarity.

Diabetes management

Spinach contains an antioxidant known as alpha-lipoic acid, which has been shown to lower glucose levels, increase insulin sensitivity, and prevent oxidative stress-induced changes in patients with diabetes.

Healthy skin and hair

Spinach is high in vitamin A, which is necessary for sebum production to keep hair moisturized. Vitamin A is also necessary for the growth of all bodily tissues, including skin and hair. Spinach and other leafy greens high in vitamin C are imperative for the building and maintenance of collagen, which provides structure to skin and hair.

Iron

A lack of iron in the diet can affect how efficiently the body uses energy. Spinach is a great source of iron, along with lentils, tuna, and eggs. Make sure to combine vitamin C-rich foods with plant iron to improve absorption.

Calcium

Spinach contains approximately 250 milligrams of calcium per cup (cooked), however, it is less easily absorbed than calcium from sources like dairy products. Spinach has a high oxalate content, which binds to calcium making it difficult for our bodies to use.

Magnesium

Spinach is also one of the best sources of dietary magnesium, which is necessary for energy metabolism, maintaining muscle and nerve function, heart rhythm, a healthy immune system, and maintaining blood pressure. Magnesium also plays a part in hundreds more biochemical reactions that occur in the body. Spinach's antioxidants also protect skin, eyes, and oral health by protecting from tooth decay and gum disease or infections. They also protect against more serious conditions including free radical damage, which can result in heart disease, cancer, autoimmune responses, and cognitive disorders.

Eye Health Spinach nutrition contains vitamin A in the form of carotenoids, which benefit eye sight by preserving the health of the retina, macula, and cornea. Two of spinach's carotenoids called lutein and zeaxanthin are primary antioxidants needed to prolong eye health, especially as someone ages.

Spinach is correlated with decreasing the risk for age-related eye disorders including macular degeneration. For example, zeaxanthin found in spinach works to filter out harmful light rays from entering the cornea. And spinach's other carotenoids protect vulnerable tissues of the retinal area from oxidative stress that can result in blindness, cataracts, and other complications.

High Source of Magnesium

According to researchers, spinach is one of the best sources of magnesium. And very importantly the magnesium in spinach stays intact after being cooked too. (11) Magnesium is a vital nutrient within the body that contributes to overall cellular health and plays a part in more than 300 different bodily functions. Unfortunately however, many adults in developed nations are actually experiencing a magnesium deficiency – and most aren't even aware of it.

Magnesium is needed to regulate calcium, potassium, and sodium which together all control neuromuscular signals and muscle contractions. This is why a magnesium deficiency can sometimes result in muscle pains and cramps. Magnesium deficiency is also associated with insomnia, mood disturbances, headaches, high blood pressure, and an increased risk for diabetes. It's incredibly easy to add more spinach to your diet – use it in smoothies and juices, add it to scrambled eggs, make a spinach salad, use it as a pizza topping.

Coconut oil Coconut oil is the only alkaline forming oil. It contains healthy fats known to benefit the body, rather than harm it. Experts recommend using raw, virgin coconut oil as a replacement for vegetable oils that are chemically processed.

Help Maintaining Your Skin PH

Our skin loves coconut oil a lot because coconut oil's medium-chain fatty acids are very similar to those contained in our skin oil. For that reason, our skin is able to maintain its pH level at below 5.0 with coconut oil. Maintaining at such acidity helps to block invasion by harmful bacteria and other destructive microorganisms.

By killing harmful germs that attack your cells and stopping free radical reactions that destroy your tissues, your cells are able to restore its metabolism. But coconut oil benefits your skin even more by boosting that metabolism further.

Clinical studies have shown that coconut oil has anti-microbial and anti-viral properties, and is now even being used in treating AIDS patients. Studies conducted in the Philippines last year showed that coconut oil does indeed reduce the viral load in AIDS patients.

Once mistakenly thought to be bad because of its saturated fat content, coconut oil is now known to contain a unique form of saturated fat that actually helps prevent heart disease, stroke, and hardening of the arteries.

The saturated fat in coconut oil is unlike the fat found in meat or other vegetable fats. It is identical to a special group of fats found in human breast milk that have been shown to improve digestion, strengthen the immune system, and protect against bacterial, viral, and fungal infections. These fats, derived from coconut oil, are now routinely used in hospital IV formulations and commercial baby formulas. They're also used in sports drinks to boost energy and enhance athletic performance.

Coconut oil has been used throughout Asia and the Pacific for thousands of years as both a food and a medicine. Even today it holds a highly respected position in the Ayurvedic medicine of India. Only recently has modern medical research confirmed the many health benefits traditionally attributed to this remarkable oil.

Another incredible fact about coconut oil is that even though it is a fat, it actually promotes weight loss! The reason is again because of the healthy medium chain fatty acids. These fatty acids do not circulate in the bloodstream like other fats, but are sent directly to the liver where they are immediately converted into energy, just like carbohydrates. So the body uses the fat in coconut oil to produce energy, rather than be stored as body fat. Medium chain fatty acids found in coconut oil also speed up the body's metabolism, burning more calories and promoting weight loss. The weight-loss effects of coconut oil have been clearly demonstrated by many researchers. They offer wonderful health benefits and are nowhere found more abundantly in nature outside coconut oil. For the hypothyroid sufferer the medium chain fats rev up the body's sluggish metabolism and promote weight loss as well.

What is the first thing that comes to mind when you hear "fatty acid"? Chances are you think of dangerous, artery-clogging fat. But is this really true?

The truth is, we need fat in order to survive. We need essential fatty acids for brain function, a healthy immune system, and the production of hormones. The problem is not all fats are the same. Hydronated oils such as canola, corn and soy are filled with dangerous trans-fats and processed with toxic solvents that are commonly added to packaged foods.

On the other hand, medium-chain triglycerides (MCTs), also known as medium-chain fatty acids, make up 64% of coconut oil.

Teeth and Gums

Coconut oil pulling has been used in Ayurvedic medicine for more than 3000 years. It works by pulling the toxins and bacteria out of the gums. Bacteria found in the gums is a major cause of plaque, gum disease and gingivitis.

Watermelon

Watermelon has a pH level of 9.0, which means it's very alkaline. It's also 92% water, so it's super hydrating and thirst quenching, and it is an excellent source of vitamin C, lycopene, and beta-carotene. Researchers have studied lycopene and other individual plant compounds in watermelon for their anti-cancer effects.

Although lycopene intake is linked to a lower risk of some types of cancer, the results are mixed. The strongest link so far seems to be between lycopene and cancers of the digestive system. Lycopene appears to reduce cancer risk by lowering insulin-like growth factor (IGF), a protein involved in cell division. High IGF levels are linked to cancer. Lifestyle factors, including diet, may lower the risk of heart attacks and strokes by reducing blood pressure and cholesterol levels.

Several nutrients in watermelon have specific benefits for heart health.

Studies suggest that lycopene may help lower cholesterol and blood pressure. It can also help prevent oxidative damage to cholesterol. Watermelon also contains citrulline, an amino acid that may increase nitric oxide levels in the body. Nitric oxide helps your blood vessels expand, which lowers blood pressure.

Other vitamins and minerals in watermelon are also good for your heart. These include vitamins A, B6, C, magnesium and potassium. Watermelon may help lower inflammation and oxidative damage, since it's rich in the anti-inflammatory antioxidants lycopene and vitamin C.

Fresh herbs

All fresh herbs are considered alkalizing. Parsley, in particular, is very rich in alkaline compounds, as is basil and dried dill weed. No matter what you choose, simply using more fresh, dried herbs in your meals is a great way to follow a more alkaline diet.

Sprinkle fresh thyme on salmon or chicken that's headed for the grill: Among fresh herbs, thyme has the second-highest amount of antioxidants (sage has slightly more), according to its oxygen radical absorbance capacity-a measure of a food's ability to fight off disease-causing free radicals in our body. Thyme is also a very good source of vitamins A and C, as well as iron and dietary fiber.

Sprinkle fresh thyme on salmon or chicken that's headed for the grill: Among fresh herbs, thyme has the second-highest amount of antioxidants (sage has slightly more), according to its oxygen radical absorbance capacity-a measure of a food's ability to fight off disease-causing free radicals in our body. Thyme is also a very good source of vitamins A and C, as well as iron and dietary fibre.

Most of us have herbs and spices in our kitchen cabinet somewhere and they often get haphazardly added to recipes and culinary creations. Interestingly, there are many health benefits of herbs and spices, not to mention they improve the taste of so many foods! The problem is, most herbs and spices have been sitting on a grocery store shelf for a long time, and thus they don't have much nutritional value left. I recommend growing them yourself whenever possible, but if you can't, always purchase high quality organic ones. All spices originate from plants: flowers, fruits, seeds, barks, leaves, and roots. Herbs and spices not only improve the taste of foods, but can help preserve them for longer periods of time. Herbs and Spices have antibacterial and antiviral properties and many are high in B-vitamins and trace minerals. True sea salt, for instance, contains 93 trace minerals. Most herbs and spices also contain more disease-fighting antioxidants than fruits and vegetables. The problem in America is that the most potent and healthy herbs are rarely used, mainly from lack of knowledge about them, while the least potent (salt and pepper) are the most commonly used seasonings.

Cayenne

Cayenne has many health benefits and can improve the absorption of other nutrients in foods. It has been shown to increase circulation and reduce the risk of heart problems. Though available in capsule form, it is also a great addition to many foods. In small amounts, it can be added to practically any dish, meat, vegetable or sauce. As tolerance to the spicy flavor increases, the amount added can be increased also.

 Basil has anti-inflammatory and antiviral properties and can help prevent osteoarthritis. It has been used in digestive disorders and is being studied for its anti-cancer properties. Though commonly used in Italian cooking, Basil is a versatile herb that can be added to practically anything. Fresh is always best, but dried is ok too as long as it is freshly dried. Basil can be sprinkled in omelets, on baked or grilled veggies, in soups, on meats or sliced fresh into salads. Layered with tomato and mozzarella cheese, it makes a wonderful Salad.

Dill Weed/Seed

Dill has antibacterial properties but is most known for its stomach settling ability (ever wonder why pregnant women crave pickles?). It contains a variety of nutrients but loses most when heated to high temperatures. For this reason, it is best used in uncooked recipes or in foods cooked at low temperatures. It is a great addition to any type of fish, to dips and dressings, to omelets or to poultry dishes.

31365189R00056

Printed in Great Britain
by Amazon